Contents

Group approaches in psychiatry

J. Stuart Whiteley, MB ChB FRCP(Ed) MRCPsych DPM
and
John Gordon, BA (Harvard)
Henderson Hospital
Sutton, Surrey

Routledge & Kegan Paul
London, Boston and Henley

First published in 1979
by Routledge & Kegan Paul Ltd
39 Store Street,
London WC1E 7DD,
Broadway House,
Newtown Road,
Henley-on-Thames,
Oxon RG9 1EN and
9 Park Street,
Boston, Mass. 02108, USA
Set in 11 on 12pt Imprint 101 Series by
HBM Typesetting Ltd,
Chorley, Lancs.
and printed in Great Britain by
Redwood Burn Ltd,
Trowbridge and Esher

British Library Cataloguing in Publication Data

Whiteley, J Stuart
Group approaches in psychiatry.—(Social and
psychological aspects of medical practice).
1. Group psychotherapy
I. Title II. Gordon, John III. Series
616.8'915   RC488   78-40462

ISBN 0 7100 8970 8

Acknowledgement

We are indebted to Mrs Peggy McCarthy for her patience and perseverance in translating the manuscript into typescript.

Introduction

Our book attempts to cover the field of group interaction in psychiatry. We look at small, large and specialised groups, not only for their treatment potential but also for the way that groups determine the course and mode of interpersonal activity.

Human life is group life, and mental illness becomes manifest in the group situation when we have to relate to, communicate with and respond to the expectations of others.

The book is largely a review of the field and in some instances a review of reviews. We can draw upon our personal experiences and research findings and present original data and thought in certain areas where we may have had the opportunity to achieve an extra dimension of experience, e.g. the *therapeutic community*, but this is not the primary aim of the book. Instead, we are trying to present to the trainee psychiatrist, social worker, nurse or other aspiring group worker in the mental health professions a summary of what he should know about group work in psychiatry.

We deliberately draw upon both the psychological and the sociological areas of knowledge and exploration because of our belief in the social basis of mental illness. Above all, we hope that the book is a practical guide to what happens in a group and how to channel what happens into a beneficial therapeutic course.

The living group

I

'Why a group ?', asks many a patient to whom group therapy is suggested. 'I'm ill and I want to see a doctor, not people who are as bad as I am.'

We live and work in groups and find in our personal interactions with others sources of emotional satisfaction and growth. Throughout our lives we are subjected to the demands and the pressure of groups, both small and large, from the family to society in general, and we are ill-equipped to survive without the co-operation of and contact with fellow human beings. Human behaviour in the group is different from the behaviour of the individual alone or in a dyad. In the group we have to be aware of and respond to the cues and signals of a number of other people. We have to compromise and abandon our own egocentric needs in order to maintain our place in the group, but at the same time group membership offers us strength and support. Major threats, such as loss of employment or even loss of life, can be faced and overcome by the group that bands together to institute a work-in or mobilises its resources to withstand a siege or bombardment. Indeed, the threat from outside is one of the most powerful incentives to group formation and cohesion. The strengths and the resources of such a group, however, do not rest on its material attributes alone but to a great extent on the emotional fervour that is engendered by group participation. This fundamental two-level quality of group life and functioning is one that pervades all considerations of group behaviour.

Social behaviour in groups

The study of group behaviour (Le Bon, 1895) took root in the latter part of the nineteenth century and was initially based on observations of crowd phenomena. Freud (1921) introduced into this descriptively accurate work his developing psychoanalytic theories, and social scientists began systematically to investigate group structure and processes. Gradually two streams of major enquiry evolved – a group *analytic* and a group *dynamic* course.

Long before this, the particular qualities and behavioural propensities of the crowd had been, at least implicitly, recognised and put to use by powerful leaders in the military, political, religious and revolutionary fields. Wesley was one who stirred large congregations to confession of their sins and conversion to God by playing on the suggestibility, dependency, primitive fears and the need to belong which the large group engenders. The mobs of the French Revolution were stirred by manipulative leaders into violent behaviour that, as individuals with a personal responsibility to bear, few of them would have contemplated.

Nearer to our own times, the mass rallies of the Nazi leaders similarly utilised all the factors that would induce the individual to abandon his self-control and critical judgement to the power of the group. Ritualistic behaviour, slogans to chant, uniforms to wear and colours to carry, all draw the individual into the mass identity of the group which seems above individual responsibility and guilt in its pursuit of 'the cause'. The projection of all that is bad on to the outside—in this case the Jewish race—finally unifies the group against the alleged threat from without, and the charismatic leader can mould the group's forces at his will and to his own purpose.

While these examples illustrate the manipulation of group forces by the leader, we can also see how membership of the group gives to the individual a vital force that may otherwise be lacking from his individual existence.

Each generation throws up its cult or fashionable clique around which, in particular, young people who lack a secure identity or feeling of well-being and purpose will gather with enthusiasm. In the United Kingdom to some extent the armed forces provided such a group identity during and immediately after World War II. Following this period, but in a less socially acceptable way, Teddy Boys, Skinheads and Rockers in their turn provided the common uniform, the in-group behaviour, the mutual support of the membership and the illusion that whatever the group did was above, or not answerable to, the dictates of individual conscience or wider social values.

The phenomenon of football fan violence illustrates the fragility and vulnerability of individual intentions when confronted with the influence of group forces, particularly the automatic compliance that is typical of large groups that lack strong leadership. Historically, football supporters have been promoted by the clubs as a 'good' thing, both for the team and for the benefits that membership of a social group can give to people with otherwise featureless lives. The colours, the songs and chants and the competition with rivals have been fostered with good intent, but, without clear leadership from above, subversive secondary leaders have taken over and diverted the ready-made mobs to their own purposes of violence, excitement and social disturbance, in a way that has little or nothing to do with the parent club.

The study of mass behaviour

It is this loss of self-responsibility and surrender to a mob rule that particularly caught the attention of the early observers. Le Bon (1895), whom Freud quotes extensively and with respect, clearly sets the scene, and we can do no better than begin with a summary from Freud's own account in *Group Psychology and the Analysis of the Ego* (1921). Le Bon remarked upon the fact that when individuals are transformed into a group they are 'put in possession of a sort of collective mind which makes them feel, think and act in a manner quite different from that in which each individual of them would feel, think and act if he were in a state of isolation'. Le Bon explained this transformation in terms of the emergence in groups of a racial unconscious, a substratum of inherited characteristics which imbues every individual thought, feeling and action with an average quality. He describes group behaviour as barbaric, impulsive, changeable and ruled by fantasy. The group has a sense of omnipotence, reacting in extremes, simply but with exaggerated feelings and excited only by excessive stimuli.

The members act on instinct like a child or primitive being. At times contradictory ideas may exist and be tolerated side by side. Freud believed that group membership merely provides the conditions under which the individual could throw off the repressions of his unconscious impulses, and that the different behaviour that results is due to the expression of these unconscious drives. While Le Bon considers the heightened susceptibility and contagion of group behaviour as a form of hypnosis, Freud attributes

3

the uniformities of group life to the basic similarity of the under-lying unconscious drives which are now given outlet.

Jung (1936), incidentally, makes several references to the same primitive phenomena in the mass which he also attributes to unconscious drives and archetypal functioning: 'A gentle and reasonable being can be transformed into a maniac or a savage beast and one is always inclined to lay blame on external circum-stances but nothing could explode in us if it had not been there' (Jung, 1938).

Freud notes, however, that the concepts of contagion, hypnosis and suggestibility—'The conditions under which influence with-out logical foundation takes place'—must themselves be analysed. At this point in the argument, Freud introduces his principal contribution. 'We will try our fortune, then, with the supposition that love relationships (or to use a more neutral expression, emotional ties) also constitute the essence of the group mind.' In effect, Freud postulates that, psychologically, group formation is the result of the mutual identification of members with one another on the basis of their love for the leader (or for certain ideas and values). This love is a derivative of the early libidinal relation-ship between child and parent and as such is the emotional foundation not only of mutual identification but of the suscepti-bility and voluntary obedience of group members to the will of the leader. Loss or absence of the leader can lead to panic and disintegration of the group, and Freud mentions the collapse of the German army in 1918, primarily because the officers neither merited nor nourished the libidinal ties between themselves and the soldiers in the field.

The two features of group behaviour that Le Bon and other observers emphasise are the inhibition of intellectual functioning and the heightening of affectivity. But Freud also refers to evidence that the 'group mind' is capable of more productive work and cites the development of language, folklore and the general stimulus that a social group may give to an individual who then goes on to achieve intellectual or cultural accomplishments. Indeed, Freud distinguishes between short-lived groups—e.g. a revolutionary group, which might have just the dramatic qualities that Le Bon recounts—and stable, more organised groups in normal society. Since leadership is a crucial factor, Freud pays particular attention to the role of the leader in large social groups such as the church and the army. Subsequent theoretical writings on group psychotherapy stress these same fundamental aspects of groups, i.e. intense emotional involvement with a corresponding intellectual deficiency unless clear leadership directs the vast group energies into productive channels.

Despite his awareness of group phenomena, Freud did not utilise the group in psychiatric treatment, perhaps because his major interest lay more in the further elaboration of psychoanalysis as a scientific psychology and as a research instrument for the study of intra-psychic functioning. In *Group Psychology and the Analysis of the Ego* he is directing his attention to the wider aspects of society rather than to the small group as we would know it today. However, there were, even in the 1920s, a small number of psychoanalysts, headed by Trigant Burrow, who did come to see the possibility of analysis in a group setting. Burrow (1926a) took the view 'that it was futile to attempt to remedy mental disease occurring within the individual mind as long as psychiatry remains blind to the existence of mental disease within the social mind'. Burrow, with his students, founded the Lifwynn Foundation in 1927 to further study this possibility, but the practice of *treatment in groups* was slow to develop (see chapter 2).

The study of group dynamics

The study of *group behaviour*, however, was gradually refined and moved from descriptions of the crowd to more theoretical and scientifically designed explorations of everyday social groups.

One of the first social psychologists to move into the field was William McDougall, whose thesis in *The Group Mind* (1920) asserted the reality of a group mind independent of the individual group members. His work was critically received, but nevertheless provoked considerable debate. F. H. Allport, McDougall's leading antagonist, exposed 'the group fallacy' (1924, quoted in Mills, 1962):

> alike in crowd excitements, collective uniformities and
> organised groups, the only psychological elements are
> discoverable in the behaviour and consciousness of the specific
> persons involved. All theories which partake of the group
> fallacy have the unfortunate consequence of diverting attention
> from the true locus of cause and effect, namely, the behavioural
> mechanism of the individual . . . If we take care of individuals,

5

psychologically speaking, the groups will be found to take care of themselves.

McDougall's analysis, however, was more than an exercise in mystical reification. He stressed the factor of organisation in groups and listed five principal conditions of organisation:

1 some degree of continuity of existence in the group for some time, either material (the same individuals stay in the group), or formal (a number of individuals occupy a system of fixed positions);

2 the members must have some idea of the nature, composition, functions and capacities of the group so that an emotional relationship to the whole group evolves;

3 the group must interact with other groups;

4 the group should have customs, traditions and habits, especially those that regulate inter-member relationships; and

5 the group should have a definite structure reflecting the specialisation and differentiation of functions of its constituents.

Freud, who quoted McDougall (1920) in *Group Psychology and the Analysis of the Ego* (1921), interpreted McDougall's concept of organisation as an attempt to equip the group with the attributes of the individual, particularly of the *ego*. But McDougall's emphasis on group structure, and the implication of his third condition that groups exist in a wider environment, provided a theoretical framework within which a group-level concept, such as a group goal, could be logically derived without neglecting the existence of individual group members (see the discussion of Mills and of Cartwright and Zander on the group goal in chapter 3).

The dispute within social psychology over the nature of groups led to the production of research evidence (Hunt, 1964) that accounted for the common attitudes, beliefs and goals attributed to a group mind in terms of processes of communication in groups (Allport, 1920, 1924, 1934; Jenness, 1932a, 1932b; Bernard, 1924); conformity-inducing pressures (Dickens and Solomon, 1938; Dudycha, 1937; Harvey, 1935); sympathy (Mead, 1934); imitation (Miller and Dollard, 1941) and suggestibility (Hull, 1933).

Four studies were particularly influential in setting the foundation for subsequent *group dynamics* research.

Informal norms and task effectiveness

An important series of investigations was carried out between 1927 and 1932 by Mayo at the Western Electric Company's Hawthorne Works in Chicago (Mayo, 1933; Roethlisberger and Dickson, 1939). The term *'Hawthorne effect'* derived from some unanticipated findings, in groups of workers subjected to experimental conditions, that no relation existed between any manipulation of the experimental variable—e.g. the level of illumination in workshops—and industrial production. Rather, a worker's productivity increased in the experimental groups even when illumination was decreased, dropping only when the light became so dim that no one could see properly. Increased production was therefore attributed to 'the changed social situation of the workers, modifications in their level of psychological satisfaction, and new patterns of social interaction, brought about by putting them into the experiment room and the special attention involved' (Etzioni, 1964).

The major finding of Mayo's research was the significance of social factors and, in particular, of group membership. The amount of work carried out by any individual worker was set by social norms, not physiological capacity. Non-economic rewards and sanctions, such as the affection and respect of colleagues, affected a worker's behaviour and could limit incentive plans. Also, workers held beliefs about the minimum work required of them so as not to endanger their jobs and about the maximum they could produce before pay rates might be reduced. These beliefs regarding the expectations of management were found to be objectively untrue, but they nevertheless influenced the group norms for production. As group members,

> each individual did not feel free to set up for himself a
> production quota; it was set and enforced by the group.
> Workers who deviated significantly in either direction from
> the group norms were penalised by their co-workers.
> Individual behavior is anchored in the group. A person who
> will resist pressure to change his behavior as an individual
> will often change it quite readily if the group of which he is a
> member changes its behavior [Etzioni, 1964].

The experimental creation of social norms

Sherif (1936) designed a rigorous laboratory experiment to investigate the *autokinetic effect*, based on comparisons between an individual's perceptions alone and in the company of two or three others. The autokinetic effect is easily created by presenting a point of light to a person in complete darkness when he will see the light appearing in different places in the room each time. This is not an artificial phenomenon but results from the fact that 'in a completely dark room a single point of light *cannot* be localised definitely, because there is nothing in reference to which you can locate it' (Sherif, 1936).

Sherif was primarily interested in two problems (1936):

(1) What will an individual do when he is placed in an objectively unstable situation in which all basis of comparison, as far as the external field of stimulation is concerned, is absent ? And (2) What will a group of people do in the same unstable situation ? Will the different individuals in the group give a hodgepodge of judgments ? Or, will they establish a collective point of reference ? If so, of what sort ? If every person establishes a norm, will it be his own norm and different from the norms of others in the group ? Or will there be established a common norm, peculiar to the particular group situation and depending upon the presence of these individuals together and their influence upon one another ?

Sherif, in fact, found that an isolated individual developed a range of judgements as to the perceived movement of a point of light and within that range established a reference point (norm or standard) that was peculiar to the individual. Successive judgements were given within the range and in relation to the subjective reference point. Once a range and point of reference were established, they tended to persist over second and third trials of 100 judgements. The ranges and norms of individuals varied.

On the other hand, when individuals for the first time faced the situation as group members, a range and standard within the range were also established that were specific to the group. 'If, for the group, there is a rise or fall in the norms established in successive sessions, it is a group effect; the norms of the individual members rise and fall toward a common norm in each session,' writes Sherif. To the possible objection that the group norm was merely the leader's norm, and that the leader was uninfluenced by the other members, Sherif replied that, empirically, a leader's judgements (i.e. first judgements) were observed to be influenced eventually by those of his followers. If the leader changed his norm after the group norm was established, he ceased to be followed.

Sherif also discovered that when individuals who had first established their own ranges and norms were put together in a group, the ranges and norms tended to converge; this convergence, however, was less than if they had first worked together as a group without the opportunity to stabilise their individual norms.

Finally, once a member's group norm was fixed, and he was subsequently presented with the experimental stimulus, he perceived the situation in terms of the group range and norm instead of his initial subjective reference. Sherif's experiment demonstrated the formation of social norms and supported sociological and anthropological findings 'that new and supra-individual qualities arise in group situations'.

Social norms in a natural group

Newcomb (1943) also carried out a study of social norms, using attitude questionnaires and interviews to determine the political views of university students. The focus of this investigation was on the power of the group, in this case the university community, to effect changes in the students' attitudes. Since most entering students came from 'conservative' backgrounds, they tended to hold opinions and beliefs that differed from the more 'liberal' university atmosphere. Newcomb's data—comparisons between senior and freshman students—regularly showed that the former held more 'liberal' views, which tended to be rewarded in terms of status (selected more often to represent the university in the wider society) and good reputation (seen by others to identify more with the university).

Newcomb's study showed how conflicting group loyalties, in this case between the home family group and the university group, together affected the formation and adoption of attitudes (1958):

> In this community, as presumably in most others, all individuals belong to the total membership group, but such membership is not necessarily a point of reference for every form of social adaptation, e.g., for acquiring attitudes toward public issues. *Such attitudes, however, are not acquired in a social vacuum. Their acquisition is a function of relating oneself to some group or groups, positively or negatively* . . . in a community characterised by certain approved attitudes, the

individual's attitude development is a function of the way in which he relates himself both to the total membership group and to one or more reference groups.

Interaction and the development of informal structures

W. F. Whyte relied on his own observations of the Norton Street gang and the Italian Community Club. His participant's account of the interactions of the corner boys in an urban 'street-corner society' is one of the most readable in the small group literature. Whyte (1943) conveyed a vivid picture of the importance and functions of these groups in the lives of their members, who often remained in a group from early boyhood until their thirties:

> Home plays a very small role in the group activities of the corner boy. Except when he eats, sleeps or is sick, he is rarely at home, and his friends always go to his corner first when they want to find him. Even the corner boy's name indicates the dominant importance of the gang in his activities. It is possible to associate with a group of men for months and never discover the family names of more than a few of them. Most are known by the nicknames attached to them by the group. Furthermore, it is easy to overlook the distinction between married and single men. The married man regularly sets aside one evening a week to take out his wife. There are other occasions when they go out together and entertain together, and some corner boys devote more attention to their wives than others, but married or single, the corner boy can be found on his corner almost every night of the week.
>
> The life of the corner boy proceeds along regular and narrowly circumscribed channels . . .
>
> The stable composition of the group and the lack of social assurance on the part of its members contribute toward producing a very high rate of social interaction within the group. The group structure is a product of these interactions.
>
> The individual member has a way of interaction which remains stable over a long period of time. His mental well-being requires continuance of his way of interacting.

Whyte discerned a system of mutual obligations within the group which was vital to its cohesion and survival. Often, under-lying obligations came to light only when a relationship between members broke down. Violations of obligations were related to status, and the group leader could not fail to meet his personal obligations without jeopardising his position and causing confusion. A member's position in the gang structure determined his initiatives in proposing action for the group; a leader frequently proposed action, often relying on his subordinates to communicate with the other members, while a follower suggested action to the leader only if they were alone. Whyte's emphasis on processes of interaction and the social structure within a group influenced many subsequent studies.

Sociometry

Finally, Moreno and his associate Jennings should be mentioned, not so much for a specific study as for the invention of a technique —*the sociometric test*—that is widely used in group research. Moreno is well known for his therapeutic innovations, psychodrama and sociodrama, which he developed in Vienna and New York in the 1930s.

The sociometric test involves simply asking the members of a group to choose and reject other members in accordance with some criterion; usually members are asked whom they like and dislike the most, or with whom they would and would not like to work on a particular task. The pattern of interpersonal choice affords an insight into the formal social structure of the group.

Moreno (1951) characterised the structure in terms of the numbers of isolated members (those who neither choose nor are chosen by anyone else); unchosen members; mutual attractions (pairs); chains (linked choices, but not necessarily mutual); triangles (three mutual choices); and stars (chosen by many but chooses no one in return).

Measures of group cohesiveness have been derived from *sociograms*, diagrammatic representations of interpersonal choices, which can be subjected to sophisticated statistical and matrix algebra analysis. Moreno intended that the results of sociometric tests be used to reorganise the group by putting together people who were compatible (i.e. who had chosen each other), but this practical application of the method has rarely been used. His own experience with the test is described in Moreno's major work, *Who Shall Survive?* (1934), and ongoing research was reported in the journal *Sociometry* which was founded in 1937 (Moreno, 1941, 1947, 1954; Moreno and Jennings, 1944; Jennings, 1950).

'Why a group?'

One way of viewing mental illness would be to regard it as primarily a problem of interpersonal relationships and communications and thus depending upon social interaction for its manifestation. In a sense, then, mental illness is to some extent a group product, socially based and structured. Psychotic behaviour is characterised by unclear and disordered communications, misinterpretation of another's intentions and extensive misperception of the social environment. Neurotic behaviour, although to a lesser degree, is similarly an expression of insecurity and inadequacy in the negotiation of interpersonal encounters, while personality disorders are classically examples of gross social malfunctioning and maladaptations.

Seeing the psychiatric patient in the group or social setting is to see the 'illness' in action. Nowhere has this been applied or demonstrated more successfully than in the family when it is seen as a group entity. Rather than being deposited in one individual, the 'ailment' is seen as it affects or is contributed to by all concerned in that particular and circumscribed group, and the total group behaviour comes to represent the common emotional disturbance of the members. The rationale for group treatment is that, if mental illness is viewed as a disorder of interpersonal functioning, it may be more clearly understood and remedied through exploration, insight and readjustment in the group interpersonal context that gave rise to it in the first place.

By the mid-1930s two streams of activity in the group field— *group therapy* and *group dynamics*—were already discernible. In succeeding chapters small, large and specialised group situations are considered both as aetiological factors in mental disorders and as treatment methods. The study of group dynamics clearly has considerable application in many spheres of social life, and the development of this important branch of social science is also described. While group therapy and group dynamics often take divergent courses and have dissimilar objectives, in psychiatric practice a skilful blend of each is called for in order to achieve maximum effect in the pursuit of mental health in the social setting.

The small group as a medium for therapy

There is a certain amount of argument as to when and where group psychotherapy originated. Certainly the history of group psychotherapy is very short and there has been considerable modification during its brief life.

Instances of treatment in groups that undoubtedly invoked the naturally occurring phenomena of group life without knowledge of what was being utilised can be found in Mesmer's assembling of patients around the tub to receive the animal magnetism of the master and Charcot's treatment of hysterical patients by hypnosis which he conducted in, or before, groups of other patients. Pratt in 1907 is customarily accredited with originating group therapy in most reference books, but he also came by accident upon the group forces. He set out to teach tuberculous patients in a group how to deal hygienically with their sputum and how to live with and manage their debilitating illness. He discovered how the patients could be inspired by his own leadership and supported by each other and introduced 'thought control clinics' in which he read poetry and verses from the Bible and introduced philosophical discussions as a means of encouraging the maximisation of an individual's resources through group contagion. The method was applied to peptic ulcer patients (Chappell *et al.*, 1937), to stammerers, where the neurotic element begins to be emphasised (Greene, 1932) and to hospitalised schizophrenics (Lazell, 1921), but still in the form of didactic lectures in classroom style. Marsh (1931), a minister turned psychiatrist, also worked with psychotics using both the didactic model and what was called the 'repressive–inspirational' model of the religious revivalist. None of these ventures can be related to present-day group *psychotherapy*, which largely emerged from the work of psychoanalysts during the 1930s. They were seeking to extend their therapeutic influence, rather than to develop the group as an economic measure to treat a number of patients by one therapist, as is often alleged.

Trigant Burrow in Connecticut, who had trained with Jung, believed that the group rather than the individual should be the focus of treatment and took the advanced view that 'an individual discord is but the symptom of a social discord' (Burrow, 1926b). He coined the term *group analysis* to describe the process of investigating in a group of fellow psychologists the phenomena of group interaction in the 'here and now'. This arose out of the suggestion of a student that the analyst and the analysand should exchange roles and explore their immediate interactions together. Later others joined in, and gradually the method was extended into work with neurotic patients (Syz, 1961).

About the same time, Moreno in Vienna was working with groups and in 1932 he coined the term *group psychotherapy*. His approach was less psychoanalytic and more concerned with social interaction. Since Moreno believed that a group unconscious did not exist in the way that other psychoanalysts were beginning to affirm, he later developed the methods of psychodrama and socio-drama which focused treatment on providing reality-testing situations. Such were the first beginnings of an interest in specific group treatments in psychiatry. The different emphasis and different techniques and application of these latter two types of group approach and what was to develop from them are discussed by Meares (1973).

Psychoanalysis in groups

The decade before World War II saw the real development of psychoanalysis in groups. Slavson (1959) was probably the most influential figure to emerge from this period. He commenced group work with children in 1934, but this consisted of free-ranging group *activity*, which was largely cathartic. Later he introduced verbalisation into the groups, particularly with adolescents, and free association and the interpretation of resistance and trans-ference so that, he writes, 'the therapeutic process in groups does not differ in essentials from sound individual psychotherapy'. He then distinguished *directive group therapies* from *psychoanalytic group therapy* to describe counselling, structured discussion or activity where free association was minimal. Slavson attributed to Schilder the distinction of conducting the first group psychoanalysis with adult patients in 1934. The latter based his work on psycho-analytic principles but also focused on the interaction between the group members. In these early days Freudian theory was incor-porated into the group setting and the analyst, working with small groups of six to eight patients, would proceed much as in indi-vidual analysis, working with each patient through transference situations, uncovering oedipal guilt and infantile sexuality, inter-preting resistances and encouraging free association. Sometimes a method of 'going around' the group to each patient in turn was adopted, but whatever the practice the treatment processes were essentially worked out through interaction with the central, analyst, group leader.

Psychoanalysis of the group

During the early stages of World War II group psychotherapy took a decisive step away from the more orthodox psychoanalytic process that had so far developed. The Northfield Army Neurosis Centre, with its concentration of neurotic young adult patients and staffed by a series of largely psychoanalytically trained and orient-ated psychiatrists and psychologists (many of whom were in-fluenced by the Tavistock Clinic), became the centre for the development of the new group techniques. Bion, in particular, developed here and later back at the Tavistock Clinic his theories of group life which are described in the classic work *Experiences in Groups* (1961). Bion used the group setting rather as Burrow had done in the early days to examine the 'here and now' interactions that took place in groups. Others, notably Ezriel, adapted Bion's theories for therapeutic work with patients.

Bion first of all viewed the group as an entity, as if it were one being rather than made up of individuals, so that all references to its working would be made in terms of 'the group'. His Kleinian orientation led to a conception of the group as a part-object, which revived in members the primitive emotional relations and attendant anxieties that Melanie Klein had postulated, i.e. the schizoid-paranoid and depressive positions. At this deepest level, Bion (1955) used the phrase 'the psychotic group'. He adopted a largely passive observer role and allowed 'the group' to determine its own course of action. He describes two levels of functioning which co-exist in such a situation. At one level is the *work group*, where the group sets about its allotted task. This may be self-examination (or treatment), or may be the more everyday and mundane task of coming to a decision or agreeing upon a course of action in respect of a business or other organisation. While such a work group sets about its task at a conscious level, there is a second level of emotional functioning operative at an unconscious level and this is largely in opposition to the work group or threatening to swamp the latter and take over the energies of the group. This activity is called the *basic assumption group*, and Bion described three patterns of basic assumption activity:

(1) *Dependency*. The group adopts a dependent pattern of behaviour towards the leader, seeking to entice him into making the decisions and in this way doing the work for them.

(2) *Pairing*. The group sets up two of its members as the chosen coupling who, if properly nurtured, will 'give birth' to the solution of their problem. In this way the group again avoids the task but defends, promotes and fosters the pairing in the hope that this will provide the answer.

(3) *Fight/flight*. The group resists or refuses to engage in the resolution of the current task or will attempt to recruit the leader to direct them in a fight against external forces as a diversionary issue. Or, they will simply refuse or resist engaging in the task by alternative activity i.e., taking flight.

Essentially, the basic assumptions are defences against the primitive anxieties aroused by the experience of 'the psychotic group' and can change during the course of a group from one to another, or more complex mechanisms may be resorted to in support of one or another basic assumption. Thus members may be cast in the role of scapegoats, often as a diversionary, fight/flight, ploy; someone may assume a co-therapist role as a dependency measure, or for a time the group may be split by the conflict of two different but co-existing basic assumptions until one or the other gains precedence.

The group members thus set about their conscious task, but constantly interfering with the efficient execution of that task are the unconscious emotional drives and feelings of the members. As these feelings intrude upon the mind of one individual they are sensed by another, who may react in sympathy (the 'contagion' of Le Bon) to a greater or lesser degree, according to his 'valency' for a particular basic assumption. The unconscious ideas and forces wax and wane, become prominent or insignificant, but gradually enclose all in one or other form of consensual thinking or activity.

This relatively simple form of basic assumption group can be readily seen in any group meeting, whether 'therapeutic' or not. Jacques (1955) and Menzies (1960) have applied Bion's formulations in case studies of large organisations. The logic of Bion's theory, the absence of basic evidence to support his argument and some contradictions in the text are alluded to in a critical evaluation by Sherwood (1964), who nevertheless acknowledges the importance of Bion's work.

The development of *psychoanalysis of the group* as a whole, building on Bion's exploratory work, was particularly carried out at the Tavistock Clinic. Interest would be focused upon the group in its 'here and now' interaction and the common group tensions, aspirations, activities, fantasies and preoccupations, interpreted for the group as a whole rather than for individual members. An interpretation from a mostly passive and non-directive therapist might take the form of 'the group appears to be depending upon some super-being to come and provide the answers', when the members were protesting about the lack of information or help from the leader and their own futility and uselessness and lack of resource.

Ezriel (1950, 1967), like Bion, believed in minimal participation by the leader, interpretation to the group as a whole and a leader-centred therapy, but he placed more emphasis on the individual and interpreted individual transferences. With a non-directive, passive leader, Ezriel believed that the patient, whether in group treatment or individual therapy, would use the therapist as a screen on which to project his unconscious ideas and would manifest behaviour that illustrated three types of object relationship. First, he would try to behave in a particular way to the therapist. This is the *required relationship* and is required because the patient needs it in order to prevent the emergence of another, *avoided relationship*, which, if it was allowed by the patient to occur, would result in a *calamitous relationship*. Thus, in a first group session the individuals in the group may adopt a submissive role (the required relationship) in order to evade a natural desire to rebel against and criticise the therapist (the avoided relationship), which would result in their being turned away from treatment (the calamitous relationship which they fear). Ezriel adds to this essentially individual psychoanalytic interaction the fact that in the group the vying relationship interactions of the members will summate to a *common group tension*, which finally resolves into a *common group structure*. This is the sum of the members' relationship interactions with the leader and thus of the positions that each of them takes up in order to satisfy his own individual relationship behaviour, but at the same time to fit into the pushes and pulls he feels from the other members as they too take up their positions. The role of the therapist will then be to interpret (and Ezriel believes that interpretation is the *only* role of the therapist) first, to the group as a whole, what the common group structure seems to be in terms of the object relationship of the group as a whole, and then to the individual members, in terms of their individual object relationship and their contribution to the common group structure. The object of interpretation, without censure or other comment, is to make the patient realise that the therapist does know the content of the patient's fantasy (the avoided relationship) but nevertheless does not retaliate in the fantasised way (the calamitous relationship). The patient is thus made to compare fantasy and reality (reality-testing) and will hopefully be encouraged to dispense with the required relationship in his dealings with the leader (and others whom the leader may represent) and more openly express his real thoughts and desires; i.e., he will abandon his neurotic way of interaction.

Psychoanalysis through the group

In the preceding section we saw how psychoanalysis in the group has developed into two similar but slightly different ways of viewing the group as a whole. Bion's *group dynamic* study, which was essentially an observation of group mechanisms, has been followed up more in the field of social science than in therapy and will be taken up in the next chapter. The more *psychoanalytic* group stance taken by Ezriel and the Tavistock Clinic therapists has now been described, but a third course of action was developed out of the basic psychoanalysis in the group by Foulkes and Anthony (1957). A contemporary of Bion and Ezriel and out of much the same 'think tank', namely the Northfield Army Neurosis Unit and the London psychiatric scene immediately following the war. Foulkes, with a few early colleagues and a faithful following of students from the Maudsley Hospital in particular, steadily evolved a technique of *group analysis*, resulting in 1952 in the formation of the Institute of Group Analysis in London.

Foulkes rather straddles the gap between psychodynamic and social dynamic group theory and practice. He drew on the work of Lewin (1951) (see chapter 3) to recognise that in the group situation certain particular systems of interaction and behaviour would occur as natural phenomena and could be turned to therapeutic advantage. Thus, Lewin put forward the idea of a group as a dynamic whole operating in a social field that was made up of certain social forces (vectors) which had attracting and repelling qualities (valences). The situation is analogous to the position that iron filings may take up on a sheet of paper when a magnet is applied beneath. Patterns form and positions are taken up as the balance of attraction and repulsion holds the *status quo* in a particular way. Lewin's field theory and the study of 'group dynamics' (which was his descriptive terminology) drew attention to the concept of the group as a dynamic whole and its 'here and now' existence dependent on current forces rather than on past experience. The group has no 'childhood' to draw upon. According to Lewin's principle of contemporaneity the group's 'childhood' is contained in the present. An atmosphere is generated in the group, which is the balance of both the cohesive and disruptive forces. A *group tension* develops, which is the conflict between an individual's need and the group need. Roles are taken up and allotted. A particular type of leadership will result in a particular type of reaction from the other participants.

In group analysis cognisance is taken of this background to the group and Foulkes is dismissive of the 'group mind' theorists, quoting Lewin, who says that

> there is no more magic behind the fact that groups have properties of their own, which are different from the properties of their sub-groups or their individual members, than behind the fact that molecules have properties which are different from the properties of the atoms or ions of which they are composed. In the social field as in the physical field the structural properties of a dynamic whole are different from the structural properties of subparts. Both sets of properties have to be investigated.

Foulkes also diverges from the Bion and Ezriel psychoanalytic and leader-orientated point of view in believing that interpretations from other members of the group can be as potent and possibly more meaningful to the individual than interpretations from the leader. For the leader he envisages a rather covert role 'behind the scenes'. His attitude and behaviour are important determinants of the situation but his control is subtle and unobtrusive and for this role he is designated the 'conductor'.

The ground on which Foulkes's group analysis was worked out was Northfield and the therapeutic community therein. Although Foulkes himself withdrew after the war into small group therapy and remained to the end somewhat sceptical of his colleagues and former students' increasing interest in large groups, his psycho-social approach was a considerable influence in the further development of therapeutic communities proper as described in chapter 5. Foulkes's (1975) method of group analysis is less rigid in both theory and practice than some of the foregoing examples. In this way a more natural form of group life and interaction emerges which is readily understandable to the members but is none the less a disciplined approach to maximising the understanding of an individual's behaviour in relation to his fellows.

In *selection of the group*, an individual who would be in a minority position is excluded, e.g. a single person among married people. The members are matched for age, intelligence and general social background and given preliminary information concerning the *conditions*—they will meet in a group, i.e. as strangers, sitting in a circle—and the timing, etc., is made clear.

In the early stages of the group the members with the conductor will come to an understanding of, and agreement upon, some *principles of required conduct* such as regularity, punctuality, discretion, abstinence from out-of-group contact with each other, etc.

The conductor will largely promote the *culture of the group* by leading into a form of group free association or free-floating discussion.

This can be fostered by minimising distractions, changes or extraneous foci of interest. The room and chairs are comfortable but not rest-inducing; the pictures and curtains are neutral, and the seating pre-arranged in a circle at a uniform distance so that all may see each other. Significant interpersonal interactions occur as soon as the door opens in terms of who sits where (in relation to the conductor?), moves closer or apart. The constant situation of the room is the group analogue of the couch and encourages the emergence of free association or free-floating group discussion.

The conductor is the one person who has come to the group for a different reason from the other members. He is there and a part of the group and its interactions yet apart from the group, and his interest is in the group not the self. He is the servant of the group, setting it up, time-keeping, drawing the members back to the task if they stray over the boundary into issues that are external to the immediate concerns of the group and from his specialised position proffering interpretations and the clarification of the behaviour he observes.

The network of interpersonal communications that develops is called by Foulkes the *group matrix*. Within this the members respond in their personalised ways to the topics that are raised. An emotionally disturbing issue will provoke interest and disturbance in others until all the group perhaps is sharing in the disturbance and responding to the issue, but each in his individual way reacting from his own unconscious. This state of affairs is called *resonance*. The task of the conductor is to locate the real source of disturbance. He proceeds from the overt behaviour to the latent meaning of the behaviour. He makes the group aware of what is going on and then helps them understand why they are reacting in that way. Interpretations may be to an individual or to the group, and as the group becomes more skilled the members make more interpretations to each other and the role of the conductor can be less active. In what Foulkes terms the 'transpersonal' experience, some particular individual at any one time best represents the group preoccupations, so an individual interpretation is simultaneously directed to the group. Transference occurs to the conductor and between members but interpretations are not necessarily confined to interpretation of the transference as in strict psychoanalytic practice. Foulkes writes of the behaviour of the conductor in minimising his parent-like role but responding when help is needed in a variety of ways as '*transference analysis in action*'.

THE GROUP PROCESS

Thus far the dynamic *structure* of the group has been looked at as a whole, as the composite parts or as the pattern of interlocking pieces on the background field. Another view is seen if the group is examined in terms of its *process* or life history.

Chief among the process theorists are Whitaker and Lieberman (1965), who have described in *Psychotherapy through the Group Process* their *group focal conflict theory*. The group, once met, throws up topics for discussion and, if allowed to 'free associate', 'to take up a group structure' or 'to resonate', to borrow from the terminology of the previously described theorists, gradually begins to concentrate on a particular theme or set of ideas. The theme or set of ideas, however, bears the same relationship to the underlying group dynamic processes as the manifest content of a dream, or a symptom, bears to the latent content. In other words, it is a compromise formation. Whitaker and Lieberman analyse the latent group process into two elements. The *disturbing motive* is the shared impulse or wish of the group members, which soon engenders a shared fear or anxiety, the *reactive fear*. Essentially this view is a transposition to the group context of the psycho-analytic formulation that an id impulse (disturbing motive) conflicts with an ego or super-ego response (reactive fear), giving rise to a compromise solution. In a group, the resulting group focal conflict is largely unconscious, and progress cannot be made until the focal conflict is overcome in one way or another. The discussion waxes and wanes as either disturbing motive or reactive fear comes uppermost. As the conflict becomes more apparent—and indeed it may be a function of the therapist to clarify the focal conflict as he sees it emerge—solutions are floated by the group. These may be solutions that evade the issue, retreat from it altogether or attempt to bypass or submerge it, and will be called *restrictive solutions* since they merely restrict freedom of action and do not remove the conflict, so that sooner or later the group returns to the group focal conflict, which remains to bar its progress. Eventually an *enabling solution* may be found—and again it may be the role of the therapist to facilitate the emergence of such a solution, which provides a real answer to the problem—and the group progresses in its development. The life history of the group, and indeed the history of any one group session, will be a series of such group focal conflict situations of gradually increasing complexity, and an increasing degree of sophistication and maturity of resolution skills are shown by the group. In addition to clarifying the focal conflicts and maintaining the appropriate group culture (the range of solutions on which the group operates), the leader must help establish conditions of safety and understand each individual's contribution to the *group focal conflicts*.

The natural history of the group

There are three obvious stages to pass through in the course of a treatment group—*the opening, the ongoing task* and *the termination*. This applies both to the individual group session and to the series of meetings of an established group.

The opening of the group

The first sessions are concerned with taking stock of the situation and deciding what to do as far as the patient is concerned. Very often he overtly expresses this preoccupation by interjecting remarks such as, 'I don't know if this is the right treatment for me'. The result of such a statement is usually to halt the development of the group themes and focus attention on persuading the hesitant one to 'try a little harder'. The other patients enter into this task with such enthusiasm that one can sense in them a certain relief. There is herein a respite from the free association of the group and the worry of where it might lead. They see a tangible task to perform with something to talk about, and they can demonstrate to the therapist that they are good patients.

Each member of the group is also trying to establish an identity and a role for himself and to create a group space—indeed, the remark, 'I don't know if this is for me', is one way of doing this. There is generally little interaction between members initially, therefore, as each waits rather egocentrically for the opportunity to present his life story and problem. Again, one way of establishing his differentness from anyone else present can be to sit silently until someone is compelled to ask what he is thinking about. He may then take over the centre of conversation, to the annoyance of those who have tried to play the game by sharing the discussion and doing what they thought the therapist wanted. At this stage quite obvious similarities between the members will be denied as each wants to stick to his own specialness.

The basic reason for the member's desire to be different and special is the transference relationship between himself and the therapist which exists at some level from the moment of first encounter. At a deeper, pre-oedipal level, the transference is to the group—perhaps to the 'mother group' (Gibbard *et al.*, 1974)—and the wish to be special may mask the anxiety that, without separateness, boundaries will no longer be secure and the temptation to merge will be unleashed. Remarks are made directly to or with sidelong glances at the therapist. He is asked direct questions; any answers he may give are accepted without question on the whole, and if there is someone in the group whose initial (and at this stage superficial) transference reaction is a negative one and who dares to scorn the therapist, the group will hotly come to the defence of the latter.

If the group members were to succeed in establishing their own particular identities and accustomed roles in the group, i.e. simply to behave in the group as they had behaved on the outside, if they were able to confine the therapist to the desired role that they preferred him in so far as they were concerned, and if they were able to hold on to their differences from other people, then there would be no purpose in further treatment sessions and indeed no purpose in their seeking treatment. In all of these ways they are seeking to make their situation 'viable'. Despite their proclamations that they are dissatisfied with their lives as they stand, when treatment threatens to change those life-styles they lapse into defensive and rigidly held positions of safety where they 'know where they stand' in relationship to others.

The immediate and very real problem for the new group is to interact together. Since the basic reason why each will have sought treatment in the first place is because of problems in interpersonal interactions, they are at once faced with 'the ailment', as it were, and the way they begin to settle down into the accustomed patterns soon demonstrates the reality of the problem before the very eyes of the group.

The task of the therapist in the early stages is therefore to facilitate the process of interaction between the members. He also draws attention to the similarity between behaviour in the group here and behaviour in the social groupings outside. He may repeatedly have to remind them of the object of seeking treatment, which was to explore their interactions with others rather than avoid it, so that they could seek for more satisfying ways of interaction.

How the therapist's task should be carried out depends first upon which particular school of group treatment the therapist follows but also on which interventions make more sense to the particular group in treatment. To give a gross example, children joining together in a new activity group may be directly invited to share a toy, while adults in a sophisticated, middle-class, private therapy session are left to make their own introductions in a way appropriate to their particular social situation and conventions.

In psychoanalysis in groups it is likely that the therapist would remain largely silent and that the issue of transference to the leader would be predominant and even emphasised by the latter's apparent non-responsiveness. Feelings of abandonment and non-direction, despair, and rivalry for attention and recognition arise, and the group of sophisticated, middle-class neurotics may be able to cope with these with the gradual development of maturity and insight. A group of over-active adolescents or young adults with acting-out personality disorders may be so threatened by the seeming lack of control and support that they break down under the stress rather than rise to it; for them a more active role from the therapist with some explanation of what they are experiencing would be more appropriate.

For the therapist to be so active, reassuring and explanatory that there is no room for anxiety or uncertainty to arise, however, will kill the group as effectively as if the patients were to accomplish their search for 'viability' without challenge or confrontation.

The initial attitude of the therapist should be that 'we are meeting together to mutually explore the interaction between us'. Thus the way is left open for anything to happen, but it is indicated that all are united to pool resources, including those of the so-regarded expert, who is the paid servant of the group. Some purpose and status of respectability is also given to the group, which becomes a meeting place for the positive exploration of attitudes and behaviour rather than being seen negatively as a thrown-together bunch of social inadequates with no resources, dependent on the therapist for treatment.

How much preparatory information or theoretical explanation should be given to a forming group is a matter of contention. On the whole the psychoanalytic therapists would suggest that the minimum of information and preparation should be given in order that the process of self-examination and self-responsibility can emerge. Thus, the date, location and timing of the meeting is given but little else. Patients and indeed trainee psychiatrists may approach such a prospect with considerable apprehension, which is succeeded only by bewilderment and frustration. The engendered anxiety may even block the emergence of other issues and result in early failure.

On the other hand, an opening discourse in which the therapist lets the group know (even unconsciously) what he wants them to do sets the pattern for an unproductive support group. Rabin (1970) has reported on a variety of introductory and preparatory practices. Controlled experiments, which compared groups that were given mere basic minimal facts about time and place with groups that were given an introductory lecture (Yalom *et al.*, 1967), showed that the informed groups did best in terms of attendance, low drop-out and preoccupation with 'here and now' group activity.

At Henderson the balance is struck by giving prospective patients a brief letter which explains that 'all treatment is in groups—no individual treatment is carried out' and inviting them to a group assessment interview. Despite the seemingly adequate factual information given, some will arrive saying that they expected to see a doctor alone. The customary passive expectation of the treatment situation has thus already begun to make itself evident. The desire to see the doctor alone has overwhelmed and negated the message that they have been given that 'all treatment will be in groups' and that 'you will be seen in a group with other prospective patients', etc.

At the assessment group, which is composed of staff, present patients and other prospective new patients, reference is made to this situation as an example of 'how we will work'. The applicants are encouraged to draw similarities between themselves and others present and are asked at the end of the session if they wish to proceed with admission for treatment. At this stage, again, the determination to be passively dependent often asserts itself as some reply 'I don't know—you decide'; but a point is made of insisting that the individual himself indicate his willingness or not to enter the treatment contract.

When admission occurs, new patients attend an introductory group for the first three weeks. This was instituted in the belief that it would decrease the drop-out rate in the early stages, but it had little such effect on numbers. What it did do, however, was to improve the content and quality of the ongoing treatment.

The new patients' group has as its leader the medical director (while one of the co-therapist team is a patient from an ongoing group). Rabin (1970) remarks that, in the studies he reviewed on preparation for psychotherapy, the introductory sessions were conducted by 'a prestigious senior psychiatrist'. The group quickly and repetitively passes through the opening exchanges already alluded to, and it is largely the patient co-therapist who interjects explanatory remarks such as 'that is how it seems to you now but you'll find that what is really happening is thus . . .'. When appropriate, the therapist might give some explanation of group theory or group phenomena but this should be opportunist rather than customary. Thus if a particular incident has occurred here and now in the group, such as a hostile attack upon a new member, it can be useful to say that 'it often happens in groups that a new-comer is resented and challenged—can we try and see why this should be ?'

The introductory process is further facilitated by introducing new patients at weekly intervals over the three weeks and invoking the help of the previous week's admissions to orientate this week's admissions. The idea of the patients as mutual therapists is thus quickly accepted as a real and easily accomplished task in which to engage. The result is that when these patients join an ongoing group—although they are new patients to that group—there is already some understanding of the problems of interaction with people, and this second opportunity is entered into in a more positive way with an acceptance of the possibility of exploring feelings at a deeper level.

In the foregoing situation, of course, the small groups are but part of the therapeutic community approach (see chapter 4), whereas in the ordinary hospital or out-patient setting there may not be the same facilities for introductory group work, although a move in this direction seems worthwhile.

Drop-out from the group at Henderson was not affected by introducing the preparatory groups in terms of numbers, but a greater understanding of who dropped out and why did emerge. Thus this introductory group also acts as an extension of the selection process. Yalom (1966, 1970) studied group drop-out and records that 10 to 35 per cent of members drop out in the first 12 to 20 group therapy meetings and only after this does the group solidify. The Henderson drop-out rate is 20 per cent over the first two weeks and 31.9 per cent before the end of four weeks, i.e. over the first 20 or so small group sessions, but thereafter drop-out declines (Whiteley, 1970).

Drop-out occurs for a variety of reasons, such as resistance to change and fears of the uncertain future if neurotic defences are shed. Sometimes change will begin to take place and a marital partner or over-involved family will exert pressure on the patient

27

in treatment to leave, fearing the disturbance of the *status quo* if one member of the 'family neurosis' changes. At other times a real flight into health can occur when the group suggests to the patient that he is indeed in command of his own feelings and actions and not in the grip of an illness that can be treated only by doctors.

The ongoing group

Once the initial phase has been passed the group settles down into a cohesive whole. Dramatic incidents or acting-out behaviour becomes less frequent. Topics are repetitively mulled over and progress often seems minimal or interspersed with periods of setback. The preoccupations of the group centre increasingly upon the 'here and now' of the interactions within the group meeting and the clash of personalities, attitudes and opinions within that setting. Transference relationships predominate, as for each member the group leader, the other members and the corporate body of the group itself take on the images of key figures or object relationships in the individual's life. With the experience of a transferred relationship from an outside and possibly past real relationship to a fantasised relationship in the group comes the undercurrent of sexuality, usually infantile in its origins but complicated in the present by the impingement of adult reasoning and awareness. How deeply and safely the group and its members can go into the exploration of their emerging feelings, which hitherto will have been obscured by 'symptoms' or avoided by 'acting-out' behaviour, will depend on how much trust and support the members feel for each other. As trust increases defences are lowered, feelings are allowed to emerge, and for the therapist the task is now to help the individual make sense of the 'here and now' experiences in terms of past behaviour and future expectancy. At first, positive feelings dominate the scene. This is not to say that expressions of feeling towards the leader or the other group members are necessarily positive at a spoken level. It may well be that the individual covers up his warm feelings (for fear of what might happen if he expressed them), but his behaviour is dominated by the presence of the warmth for and desire of warmth from the other. Later the more feared negative feelings begin to make their presence felt, and now the trust in and support from the other group members is of even more importance. The hostile, angry, jealous, envious and suspicious feelings that the individual has transferred on to the group, its members and particularly its leader now seek expression. Gradually, positive and negative, good and bad aspects of the relationships are brought into some perspective. Transference is beginning to be replaced by reality, and at this stage the leader may commence to withdraw from more active participation in the group. The other group members will have become very skilled at ongoing therapy and the group can be steered towards dissolution.

The termination of the group

One group therapist has suggested that from the first meeting the group should be preparing for the end. In that life is a series of relationships that flourish only to be broken as parents die, schools are left behind and friends may move away, the severance of close relationships traumatically but repetitively repeats the pattern of infantile emotional experience and separation from the mother's body. It would be ideal if all members of the group were to work together towards dissolution, and in some out-patient groups this is a possibility with the members agreeing a time several sessions hence when they will separate. More commonly, the group holds together until one or more members begin to express wishes to terminate. These may be denied by the others and ranks may close in an effort to keep the membership unchanged, but if there are some departures then others may begin to think about leaving too and it may be wise for the therapist to propose a closure date to work towards. Ahumada (1974, 1976) has described the arrangements and some typical group processes in time-limited group psychotherapy. Not uncommonly, one or two of the group members have not 'made it' at the end of the period and feel even more bereft and hopeless as the promised new world dissolves around them. Sometimes they can form the core of a new group, but often they cannot involve themselves so readily in the novel experiences that the newcomers are working through and are probably best dealt with by individual treatment.

Ways of leaving the group can be planned and worked through as outlined above but sometimes there is an acted-out departure. Thus at Henderson, while patients who were seen as successful at follow-up would have gone through a planned departure stage, there were also those whose break-away from the group was erratic and at first sight negative. They would miss groups, break rules and generally misbehave in a way that resulted in them being discharged. (This of course refers to an in-patient treatment group.) Nevertheless, at follow-up this latter type of departure was not much less indicative of a successful outcome than was a planned departure (Whiteley, 1970). In other words, making it impossible to be allowed to continue in the relationship was in fact a way of being able to leave. 'I can't leave—you'll have to discharge me' would sometimes be said by patients who, nevertheless, departed in good spirits once told to go.

A different result was seen in those patients who abruptly disappeared without discussion, notice or a word of farewell. These were the ones unable to become fully involved at either a positive or a negative emotional level, and they were soon in difficulties again after leaving the group.

The course of an individual group session

The course of an individual group session is a miniature representation of the overall series and should be viewed in its three phases: (1) *the opening*, in which tentative ideas are floated and remarks made, usually with one eye on the therapist to see what topic or direction may please him; (2) the *main thesis* of the group, in which the members become engaged with each other and the therapist exerts his conductor role; and finally, (3) the *termination*, in which, again, the members often look to the leader to 'sum up', make them secure or otherwise control their emotional lives until the next meeting.

For the group leader, then, it is important to be able to shift between these expected roles, not necessarily responding at once to the apparent needs and demands of the group but being aware of what is desired at any one time and facilitating the gratification of that need through the resources of the group itself. In the opening stage the leader is listening and looking for the common group theme and helping the group to clarify its real preoccupation. As this emerges the work of the group begins, facing and retreating from the problem, avoiding issues and defending against the emerging fears or anxieties. Now the leader becomes the conductor, helping the group seek ways of resolving the conflict rather than providing solutions. In the terminal stage there will often be a rush of new material and a pressure of words and ideas as if the group feels that all its problems can quickly be resolved in this very session and that the session should be prolonged to meet this need. Ideas have been stimulated and feelings aroused. The role of the therapist is to indicate that at another session solutions may be found and that some uneasy feelings may have to be carried until that time. The summing-up procedure is not a good one, for it rather presumes that the leader understands everything while the group does not. Rarely, however, it may be important for the therapist to intervene reassuringly at the end of a disturbed group or with a particularly disturbed patient rather than leave anxiety precariously high in the unsupported time between sessions.

Ground rules for group therapy

Some basic rules for the group should be worked out and accepted in a contractual way by the members. These need not be extensive and may evolve in the early meetings by mutual agreement. Thus, a new member may want to move around, touch people or convert a discussion group into an encounter-type group. Some agreement on behaviour should be reached, in which the therapist also says what he is willing to do or not do, and the deviant member should then concur or leave. Time is important in psychotherapy. A fixed time period for the group should be set and not altered by anyone— least of all the therapist—unless there is some very extraordinary reason. The members will gear their thoughts and actions to the expected period of the group session. Lateness, absence or earliness all then take on significant meaning. A usual time for an out-patient group session is about one-and-a-half hours, but for an in-patient session, where the patients remain in contact between the more frequent group sessions, some time less is feasible, though never less than an hour. It takes time for the group themes to emerge and, as we have seen, there may be a desire to prolong the session by a rush of ideas at the end. Punctual termination is just as important as a punctual start, otherwise the members may feel they can always delay a little longer before coming out with the problem. Just as lateness or absence has meaning for a patient, so has it meaning for the therapist, who must as punctually stick to his obligations if he is to leave the group free to work in the 'here and now' and not be hamstrung by the feelings provoked and the uncertainty engendered by his apparent commitments else-where. Sometimes, in an out-patient group, a time limit may be set for the series, e.g. once a week for two years with an agreed holiday period when meetings will be suspended. This structuring prompts and enables the group to get on with its business and not, as in therapy with no definite time scale, keep things back later and later in the hope that somehow the more propitious time for disclosure will emerge.

In practice, however, groups can seldom proceed through a two-year life history without changes of membership. Such a group would be called a *closed group* and, hopefully, would proceed in uniform progress to maturity. More often there is an intermittent fall-out so that new members have to be admitted in what is described as a *slow-open group*. As numbers decline the therapist may suggest that new members join and he will discuss this with the group. There will be resistance to be dealt with, for a newcomer is an interloper, untrustworthy; a stranger who may steal or destroy or take over the place that an established member has won for himself in the group and particularly with the leader. On the other hand, someone at odds with the present group may see in the newcomer an ally, a saviour or a new victim to become the foil of the group. The integration of the new member is therefore a difficult and emotion-laden situation for all concerned and one with great treatment potential.

In the out-patient group it is usually suggested that patients do not interact outside the group, should address each other in terms of equality but relative anonymity, such as Tom, Mike, Mary, etc., and should not identify themselves too closely with their reality background. Thus, Tom remains Tom who works in an insurance office rather than Tom Smith who works for Simpson and Co. and lives in Hampstead Lane. In this way social inhibitions and conventions, reality fears about who knows what about whom, can be minimised and more authentic 'here and now' unconscious material can emerge. Invariably, personal information does gradually accumulate, but as the group consolidates trust deepens and outside factors become of less importance. Query (1964) has demonstrated that high self-disclosure within the group tends to be positively correlated with attraction to the group. However, in the early stages some respect for the privacy of outside life may be helpful while too much self-disclosure, too soon, can be frightening for the individual and the group. Despite discouragement, meetings outside the group do occur, but if they do so it is important that the matter is brought to the group and explored and discussed for what it might mean. Such meetings might represent disobedience, sexual acting-out to provoke the parent, or pairing-off from an unhappy situation in the group.

Privileged communications to the therapist should also be disallowed but brought to the group when they occur.

Rather than start the group with a list of rules, however, it is perhaps enough that the basic time and attendance expectancy is made clear and other opportunities are then taken to explore the pros and cons of the various expected situations as and when they arise. The therapist will usually be asked his opinion, and he can give it and explain why he feels that there should be no private communication, for instance, and invite the group to consider the position and come to an agreement.

Co-therapists in the group: leadership roles

In the psychoanalytic group the therapist will be the only non-patient member and treatment is largely leader-orientated. In the group-analytic setting of Foulkes, and in the more socially orientated groups of the therapeutic community, it is acceptable for the leader to work with a co-therapist. Yalom (1970) believes that the co-therapists should be of equal status and experience, otherwise the differential leads to tension and conflict which the group may then exploit. While the male and female co-therapists naturally fall into expected parental roles for the group, it is usual that two therapists of the same sex will also take up complementary roles and attitudes, one being more direct and confrontative, perhaps, and the other more supportive. For new therapists the presence of a colleague to monitor their behaviour or to help and support if they are under attack by the group is a real advantage. At Henderson where there can be more than one co-therapist in the group the differential status has not been found a problem. Indeed, it seems to us that two therapists of equal status would be more likely to come into conflict than an established group leader and a trainee. The advantage of the latter arrangement is that the trainee can often see things from another point of view—he may be nearer the patient's age or social situation than the established psychiatrist, for instance, and can give a valuable feed-back of his perception of current behaviour to the group leader. Conflict, or even the expression of differing ideas by the co-therapists, is however a situation fraught with danger for the group. If there are marked differences these should be worked out in staff sessions and not before the patients. It is sometimes argued that patients can profit by seeing the adult way in which their therapists can settle differences, but more commonly dependent patients are considerably disturbed by observing what they experience as the instability of their fantasised transference ideals, and it is not unknown for therapists to behave in a highly neurotic way when under stress themselves.

Some successful co-therapy teams are husband and wife, but, while giving an apparent model of a mutually satisfying relationship to the patients, such a partnership invites personal attack, splitting and testing out in a way that would be less evident in non-personally related couples, and it puts the actual relationship under considerable stress, while even inviting the group to engage in a diversionary side issue. The husband-and-wife team could be seen as a rather provocative challenge to the patient unable to make relationships and denied the reality of trying to make one here by the ground rules of the group.

Selection of patients for group therapy

Patients have to be selected for group treatment as for any other treatment in psychiatry. There is an argument for having a 'balanced aquarium' of different personality types and problems so that the group interactions may simulate real-life experience and expectations, but there is also a case for having patients with obvious similarities in the group together so that identifications can more easily be made. The problem with the balanced aquarium is that the more vulnerable personalities may go to the wall and defences be reinforced, whereas the problem with a too-similar grouping is that the patients are unchallenged in their neurotic behaviour. The compromise is that members with relatively similar *levels of maturity* should be gathered in the one group so that all can share in the interaction on equal terms. Since group psychotherapy is a verbal and reasoning interchange, comparable levels of intelligence are an important factor. Social class, marital status, sex or occupation are of less importance, and some admixture is advantageous in order to get a variety of opinion and reaction.

Locke (1961) considered the selection problem in a very commonsense manner:

> Groups are established by balancing active and passive patients, or balancing diagnostic category, or personality

characteristics, or whatever else the therapist regards as decisive. . . . The guiding factor is communication. . . . If the spread is too great between group members in any characteristics . . . if there is no common meeting ground because of the difference, there can be no communication and therefore no interaction.

Intelligence, however, sets the level at which ideas can be conceptualised in the group while the level of maturity determines the pattern of emotional expression and outlet. A patient may be disadvantaged by lack of intelligence or be excluded from the group because the immediacy of his infantile needs has no place in the more sophisticated symptom formation of more mature but still emotionally disturbed fellows.

With broad selection into comparable groupings for both levels of intellectual capacity and maturity of behavioural expression, groups can be formed to tackle a wide variety of psychiatric disorders. Thus, while one tends to think of group psychotherapy for the neurotic, groups of psychotics, the mentally subnormal, psychopaths or drug addicts have all been described and can operate with some success. The emotional needs of the patients in the group are evidenced by their pattern of behaviour. The therapist attempts to meet those needs appropriately. Thus, a patient who describes or displays psychotic behaviour in a group of neurotics will probably be viewed with some alarm and further excluded from the interchanges in the group—which only serves to enhance the psychotic productions of his inner world. Or, in their fear of his madness, the other group members may resort to angry suppression of his ideas. A patient who described the voices and bizarre incidents of what was clearly an acute psychotic episode in a group of psychopaths at Henderson, however, was easily listened to and could be led by the therapist into considering ways in which 'voices' do arise in the head—when other stimulation is lacking, or when one is cut off from people, or if alcohol or drugs are providing noxious stimulation and interfering with perception, for instance. Furthermore, the group could be drawn into discussing the symbolic or wish-fulfilling meaning of the voices as in a dream. This was possible because bizarre, near-psychotic, infantile and regressive behaviour, the 'flash-backs' of post-drug intoxication and a rich fantasy life are part of the being of the immature personality of the psychopath whom many therapists would exclude from 'normal' group psychotherapy with a mixed neurotic group for just these reasons. One method of selection utilised for the in-patient groups at Henderson is assessment by other patients. Through an exploratory group interview the present in-patient group seeks out motivation, capacity for insight, ability to withstand confrontation or assimilate interpretations and the degree to which the newcomer can identify with the other group members and they with him. If the current group elects to admit the newcomer they then feel a commitment to persevere with him through the expected stormy period of integration into the community.

The curative factors in group therapy

Yalom (1970) has discussed at length the curative factors in group therapy and these can be summarised as follows:

(1) *Imparting of information* Many of the early group workers gave didactic lectures to their patients. Although there is much opinion-seeking and advice-giving in groups, the group affords a major informal opportunity for giving patients insight into psychic phenomena, behavioural patterns and psychological mechanisms. This then leads to awareness of and control over emotional disturbance.

(2) *Instillation of hope* The sharing of experience and the encounter with recovering patients is important.

(3) *Universality* One patient remarked after a large group, 'I thought I was unique until I heard other people describing exactly what I feel. Now I feel less cut off.' Stripped of their symptom guise, the problems that emerge in the group are very similar.

(4) *Altruism* The opportunity to give something of value to others can be as important as receiving help from fellows.

(5) *Corrective recapitulation of the family group* Without exception, says Yalom, patients enter group therapy with the history of a highly unsatisfactory experience in the first and most important group—their primary family. The group resembles a family, and the developing transference relationships, particularly with the leader, allow the early experiences to be re-explored.

(6) *Development of socialising techniques* At various levels, whether in the directive treatment of adolescents or the emergence of interpersonal activity through encouragement and permissiveness, a new social awareness and ability can develop.

(7) *Imitative behaviour* In the group, patients can benefit by observing the behaviour of other patients with similar problems and will try themselves out in a variety of different modes of behaviour, seeking an alternative to current maladaptive behaviour.

The processes by which these factors are introduced and the degree to which any one influences a particular patient are dependent on the various theoretical approaches of the therapeutic schools and the particular personality of the patient. The interaction of treatment method and personality variables make one method appropriate to one patient but ineffective or even harmful to another.

Recording the group

Keeping a documentary record of the proceedings of a group session is a useful procedure for the therapist but probably has little value for the patient, although Yalom (*et al.*, 1975) found that feeding back the therapist's written summaries in both individual and group psychotherapy was of some value to both. To some extent, the group material is repetitive as the same or related problems surface time and time again in a variety of guises and social lessons are learned and re-learned before behaviour seems to change. Nevertheless, writing a record of the group transaction in a brief form after each session helps the therapist to crystallise his ideas and conceptualise the psychopathology of the members and the processes of group functioning. If he is working with a co-therapist the making of the record acts as a learning experience for both.

The simplest record keeping is a *record of attendance* (including lateness) with a note of the group theme. Such a record can give an indication of impending drop-out and may suggest the relationship between drop-out and themes discussed or problems broached.

A more complex record, intended to be used to give information to a co-therapist or a student who may not attend every session, is Murray Cox's (1973) *group therapy chronogram*. In this, each member of the group is represented diagrammatically by a circle divided into three segments to represent the opening, the main part and the termination of the group. When the group has concluded the therapist writes into each member's circle the major communications he made in the session, placing them chronologically in the appropriate segment. Interactions between members or specific responses made to one member are indicated by arrows in that particular direction.

A less complicated but usefully informative method is to make an *information and process record*. On one side of the page the main topics broached or behaviour exhibited by each individual are logged, giving verbatim quotes which are more authentic and to the point than paraphrases. Interpretations made by the therapist are indicated by blocked brackets. On the other side of the page a formulation of the group type, process and the stages of development is made.

Training for group work

Some subjective experience in a group is a useful aspect of training and, indeed, is probably an essential adjunct to becoming a group psychotherapist. The reality of dependency on the leader, the paranoia of or around a newcomer and the hostility of the old hands to the newcomer are thus learned at first hand. At Henderson new staff join the new patients' group and are encouraged to bring forward their own problems of being new to the group in parallel with the new patients. They usually attempt to quickly align themselves on the 'non-sick' side, however, and register that they are therapists and not patients, thus defending against rather than entering into the exploration of their insecurity. The staff after-group discussions and ongoing sensitivity groups will hopefully lead them into discovering how like the patients they are in their reactions to the new situation. They too come to the group with great enthusiasm; they set out to make their presence felt in the preconceived way that they carry in from the outside world; but they are met with reserve, if not hostility, questioning if not confrontation; and some adjustment of behaviour may be sought if they are to fit into the established staff team. Enthusiasm fades, disillusion takes over, the idealisation of the unit and group therapy is tarnished. From the negative position a more balanced view is reconstructed, perspectives are gained and after some months the experiences gone through and explored in the staff groups lead to a considerable understanding of the similar experiences of the patients in the group.

While an ongoing staff sensitivity or T-group is an important factor for those engaged in group work, particularly if they are working together in the same institution, the after-group discussion between the co-therapists where such exist or a mutual discussion between therapists of contemporary groups serves a similar purpose of monitoring the therapist's behaviour and opening his eyes and mind to what may have eluded him in the group. The group is an intensive emotional experience for all concerned. It moves quickly and often covertly. The therapist must be alert in every sense to the nuances of the group behaviour but such is the heightened emotional tempo that he can sometimes be carried along unwittingly in the psychopathology of the group and some supervisory support is recommended if only in the form of a review of the group's progress, with colleagues, at regular intervals.

Summary: an eclectic approach to psychotherapy in groups

Group psychotherapy offers a variety of theoretical concepts and methods of practice. The therapist will select which ideology and practice best suit his own personality and beliefs but should be perceptive and open-minded enough to adapt his techniques to the various groups he encounters and the particular needs of, and directions taken by, the group itself. Sometimes the group will be seen to fall into a classic Bion basic assumption model and at other times the group focal conflict will proceed stage by stage throughout the group session. His own behaviour will fluctuate according to the group need, but it is important that he has some basic plan of action in mind and that the group is kept moving along this path; otherwise the group sessions simply become a way of life for the patients (and the therapist) and are totally unproductive. Visualising the group both from the point of view of its type and its process is like looking at a cloth and seeing the warp and the weft, and the interweave between the two makes up the finished article.

3 Group dynamics

The clinical perspective has lent depth to the study of groups; working towards therapeutic goals, practitioners have applied concepts from the depth psychologies, particularly psychoanalysis, to understand the phenomena that confronted them in a group context. Primarily, this involved the analysis of unconscious relationships which developed among the group members as well as between them and the therapist, on the one hand, and between them and the group as a whole, on the other. The focus was on interpretation of transference and resistance.

Yet the very idea of the group as a whole stems from a wide-ranging, interdisciplinary study of groups which is not essentially clinical or therapeutic in orientation. The fact that three of the leading theoreticians of group psychotherapy in Great Britain—Bion, Ezriel and Foulkes—centred their attention on the group in addition to the individual not only demonstrated their awareness of what came to be called group dynamics research; it also showed their strong conviction that the methods and discoveries of psychologists, sociologists, social psychologists and anthropologists working within this field might fruitfully be applied and adapted to promote greater understanding of psychotherapy groups.

Although the term 'group dynamics' was first listed in the *Psychological Abstracts* only in 1945 in connection with an article by Kurt Lewin (1944) on 'Constructs in psychology and psychological ecology'—and Lewin is considered a pioneer of both the experimental and the theoretical basis of the group dynamic approach—the body of thought to which that term applies has many sources.

Lewin himself attributed extensive interest in groups to the integrating effect that he believed World War II had on the social sciences. The war created demands and made resources available for the theoretical integration of the social sciences in response to a need for solutions to pressing problems. As the focus shifted from mere descriptions of group life to an emphasis on understanding group processes and change, the development of methodological tools for research proceeded. In effect, the group-based clinical innovations of Main (1946), Bion (1961) and Jones (1953), designed to cope with practical problems of wartime emotional breakdown and the rehabilitation of servicemen, were part of an urgent revival of concern with group influence in all areas of social life. This was reflected in the foundation of the Tavistock Institute of Human Relations in Great Britain, and Lewin became director of the new Research Center for Group Dynamics at the Massachusetts Institute of Technology.

However, the war period marked a particular historical concentration on the scientific study of groups which actually can be traced further back. Sociologists since the nineteenth century have put social groupings at the centre of their theoretical and empirical work. In fact, from a sociological point of view, the classical debate regarding the primacy of the individual or of society (the group) is meaningless. The human individual is inconceivable without the prior existence of language, prolonged dependence and nurturing, and subsequent continuing socialisation. Without group life, there could at most be only physical organisms, assuming (surely unjustifiably) that survival could be assured in the absence of organisation into groups.

Cooley (1909) referred to the decisive humanising function of the primary family group. Durkheim (1933, 1952) stressed the importance of the group for social control and for mental stability. Simmel (1902, 1950, 1955) analysed the variable of group size and distinguished between the properties of dyads and triads. One such difference is the possibility for coalitions in the triad. (For more recent research which takes as its point of departure Simmel's work see Lindsay, 1972; Mills, 1953.) Thrasher (1927) studied delinquent gangs and found that some criminal activities were readily understandable as group rather than as individual behaviour. The group initiates, trains, evaluates, justifies, maintains and protects its members in their anti-social acts. Thomas and Znaniecki (1918) wrote their classic study of the immigration of Polish peasants to the United States from the point of view of what happened to established group patterns during transition to a different social and cultural environment, and Myrdal's (1944) analysis of racial discrimination in the United States was based on the idea of intergroup conflict.

In addition to the scholarly contributions of individuals, the emergence by the 1930s of several new professions, especially in the United States, permitted researchers to draw on informed, practical group experience and afforded many new opportunities for collaborative studies. Social group workers, educationists and teachers, business, hospital and public administrators all shared a concern and an interest in developing efficient ways of using groups in their various organisations. Professionals continue to consult students of group dynamics and to make direct use of university facilities; some companies (e.g. Westinghouse, the Bell Laboratories) have expanded their own resources for conducting research into groups (Cartwright and Zander, 1968).

With such a multi-faceted history, it is not surprising that the research findings produced in the field of group dynamics are extremely diverse. Any attempt to convey the group dynamics approach to the study of groups must, therefore, resort to some method of ordering the vast amount of data that has emerged since the late 1940s and early 1950s when interest in small groups mushroomed.

The necessity for such ordering is especially obvious when the magnitude of this interest is considered. Hare, who has systematically conducted a search of the literature for articles relating to small group research, found (Strodtbeck and Hare, 1954) that in the fifty-year period between 1890 and 1939 about 355 articles appeared; whereas, in the next fourteen-year period, from 1940 until 1954 when he and Strodtbeck published the first comprehensive bibliography, over 1,000 items were published. A second bibliography was included in an important selection of readings (Hare, Borgatta and Bales, 1955) and listed nearly 600 references. Finally, Hare's latest work (1962) includes 1,385 references.

The kinds of groups that are studied in these articles vary enormously: from natural groups such as street corner gangs (Whyte, 1943), work groups in factories (Roethlisberger and Dickson, 1939), boys in summer camps (Sherif and Sherif, 1953), women in university sororities (Siegel and Siegel, 1957) and residents in housing projects (Festinger, Schachter and Back, 1950) to groups composed of subjects who may have had no prior knowledge of or relationship to one another, and were usually undergraduate students who either volunteered or took part in experiments to satisfy course requirements. In the latter studies, the groups are literally creations of the researcher, which can be manipulated and subjected to maximum experimental control (for example, Schachter *et al*, 1951; Deutsch, 1949; Bavelas, 1950; Thomas, 1957).

The subject matter of these studies has also varied greatly, with the focus shifting from channels of communication to the formation of group standards and pressures on deviant members; from the nature of group cohesiveness to measuring task efficiency; from the pattern of friendships to the exercise of power; and from the effects of size to the properties of leadership.

The inevitably frequent use of different concepts, research methodologies and techniques of measurement makes such a complex body of investigations extremely unwieldy and recalcitrant to theoretical unification. Nevertheless, and recognising that some simplification must occur, three theoretical attempts to integrate the empirical small group literature have been made which seem useful. They are by no means exclusive options; on the contrary, they often overlap and merely stress different aspects of the same phenomena. Together, they should provide the clinician with a wider view of groups.

GENERAL SYSTEMS THEORY

'Relationships thinking'

The first theory to be considered is a sociological variant of general systems theory which treats the group as a type of social system. In a sense, general systems theory itself is more a comprehensive orientation in the contemporary philosophy of science than a specific theory. Much of the influence, and indeed the name, of general systems theory can be attributed to the work of Ludwig von Bertalanffy (1956, 1962, 1968), an Austrian biologist who worked in Canada and the United States. His preoccupation with 'sets of elements standing in interaction' was not totally new. Alexander Pope's line from his 1773 *Essay on Man*, 'Observe how system into system runs—what other planets circle other suns' (quoted in Beckett, 1973), was an early expression of universal interrelatedness, which is the hallmark of general systems theory. Another early example of systems thinking was the closed universe of Newtonian physics, the clockwork reality with precisely interlocking parts moving through a pattern of linear causality. Von Bertalanffy distinguished from this machine model the dynamic open systems of biology. For mechanical predictability he substituted the idea of a steady state of balanced tension (Beckett, 1973). The universe was conceived in terms of a hierarchy of systems, each containing its sub-systems and contained in its supra-systems (Miller, 1955, 1957, 1965a,b).

'Relationships thinking' instead of 'thing thinking' (Beckett, 1973) has been employed as a framework for the organisation of knowledge in many fields (cf. Durkin, 1972) including information theory (Shannon and Weaver, 1949), theory of automata (Minsky, 1967), game theory (von Neumann and Morgenstern, 1947), decision theory (Rapoport, 1959), and cybernetics (Wiener, 1948). Von Bertalanffy believed that psychoanalysis as a psychological theory was incompatible with modern scientific concepts, but psychiatrists, analysts, and group psychotherapists have found general systems theory productive (Durkin, 1972; Kernberg, 1975; Miller, 1955, 1957, 1965a,b; Grinker, 1969; Astrachan, 1970). Despite his own assessment of psychoanalytic theory, von Bertalanffy collaborated with Karl Menninger and became an honorary fellow of the American Psychiatric Association in 1967.

Definitions of various types of system

The aim of general systems theory is to provide a means for understanding 'the nature of organisation in complex phenomena' (Durkin, 1972). A system is defined in three stages (Rapoport, 1968) as:

(1) something consisting of a set (finite or infinite) of entities (2) among which a set of relations is specified so that (3) deductions are possible from some relations to others or from the relations among the entities to the behaviour or the history of the system.

As Rapoport points out, this definition is quite general and applies to phenomena such as the solar system and language as much as to social formations. In the solar system, the entities are the sun, planets, stars, etc. The relations are described in terms of position, velocity and gravitational force; and other relations, for example Kepler's laws, are derivable from the given relations. Similarly, the entities in a language are phonemes, morphemes and sentences; the relations between them are given by the rules of syntax (Rapoport, 1968).

44

The theory of social systems has been most fully developed by Parsons (1951a; Parsons and Shils 1951; see also Buckley, 1967, 1968; Cortes *et al.*, 1974). Parsons (1968) defines system as

> the concept that refers both to a complex of interdependencies between parts, components, and processes that involves discernable regularities of relationship, and to a similar type of interdependency between such a complex and its surrounding environment. . . . [*The social system*] is generated by the process of interaction among individual units. Its distinctive properties are consequences and conditions of the specific modes of interrelationship obtaining among the living organisms which constitute its units.

Roles and intrinsic system problems

A social system, according to this definition, emerges from inter-action among people, but such interaction is not random. What makes an interaction or a relationship social is the fact that it is structured in time and place according to a role; the role rather than the individual organism is the conceptual entity of the social system. In any specific interaction between an individual and one or more others, the role organises the expectations, reciprocities and responses of the actors: 'What an actor is expected to do in a given situation both by himself and by others constitutes the expectations of that role. What the relevant alters are expected to do, contingent on ego's action, constitute the sanctions' (Parsons and Shils, 1951). Role is a complementary set of expectations and actions to be carried out in accordance with those expectations; role implies a reciprocity of expectations and sanctions.

Using the concept of role, Parsons arrives at a second formulation (Parsons and Shils, 1951):

> A social system, then, is a system of interaction of a plurality of actors, in which the action is oriented by rules which are complexes of complementary expectations concerning roles and sanctions. *As a system*, it has determinate internal organisation and determinate patterns of structural change. It has, furthermore, as a system, a variety of mechanisms of adaptation to changes in the external environment. Those mechanisms function to create one of the important properties of a system; namely, the tendency to maintain boundaries.

In this definition Parsons mentions the 'determinate internal organisation' of a social system. Such organisation is the result of responses to two fundamental problems facing all social systems: the problem of *allocation* and of *integration*. The problem of allocation arises because objects of use and value are scarce in relation to what is required to satisfy every individual's needs: 'the problem of who is to get what, who is to do what, and the manner and conditions under which it is to be done' (Parsons and Shils, 1951). Human capacities and resources, facilities for the performance of roles (including power), and rewards (prestige) must be allocated. When this problem is not successfully met—when the process of allocation impedes effective collaboration or is considered illegitimate—the social system may disintegrate. The problem of integration follows from the necessity for allocation and the internal differentiations that result (Parsons and Shils, 1951):

> A social system must possess a minimum degree of integration; there must be, that is, a sufficient complementarity of roles and clusters of roles for collective and private goals to be effectively pursued . . . for conflict among individuals and groups to be kept within bounds, the roles and role clusters must be brought into appropriately complementary relations with one another.

A final definition crystallises Parsons's analysis (Parsons and Shils, 1951):

> A social system is a system of the actions of individuals, the principal units of which are roles and constellations of roles. It is a system of differentiated actions, organised into a system of differentiated roles. Internal differentiation, which is a fundamental property of all systems, requires integration. It is a condition of the existence of the system that the differentiated roles must be coordinated either negatively, in the sense of the avoidance of disruptive interference with each other, or positively, in the sense of contributing to the realisation of certain shared collective goals through collaborated activity.

The group as a social system

One application of this sociological perspective to the study of groups has been put forward by Mills (1962). He basically accepts the Parsonian definition of a group as a self-directing, goal-seeking, boundary-maintaining system subject to internal differentiation in response to personal, social and environmental realities. He adds to this some properties of feed-back that characterise groups as information-processing systems (cf. Deutsch, 1963). Through its agents (the members), the group observes, evaluates, acts and assesses the consequences of action in the face of internal and external demands. Group agents can learn from experience to better achieve collective goals (establish a culture); they can rearrange or reconstitute the structure of the group; and they can become conscious of the characteristics of their group. Feed-back mechanisms give a group the potential for self-determination and growth, which offers individual members opportunities for gratification that go beyond those available if mere survival of the group is the main incentive for members' investment and motivational energy. By group growth, Mills refers to the development of a number of capabilities:

(1) an increase in intake of information from the external environment;
(2) a capacity to make contacts and assume responsibilities beyond its current boundaries;
(3) the flexibility to change its customs, rules and techniques;
(4) the capacity to shift to or add new goals and to suspend on-going efforts in order to consider alternatives;
(5) the capacity to further differentiate without losing collective unity and to send out resources without being depleted; and
(6) the ability to increase membership and to transmit its culture and experience to the new members as well as to other groups.

The group becomes in this view a source of experience, learning and capabilities (Mills, 1962).

The five sub-systems of a group

The focus of Mills's analysis is on the group role structure, i.e. on the group as a social system. He divides the interpersonal processes within a group into five distinct levels: behaviour, emotions, norms, group goals and group values. *Behaviour* is the overt action of a person in the presence of others. *Emotions* are the drives experienced by a person and the feelings he has about others and about what happens. *Norms* are ideas about what a person should do, feel or express. *Goals* are ideas about what a group as a collective should do. *Values* are ideas that describe ideal states or conditions for the group. On each level, an element or entity—i.e. an act, a feeling, an idea about what a member or the group itself should do or become—is interrelated with the other entities on the same level; in other words, each level is treated as a sub-system of the group with its own internal dynamics (Mills, 1962):

1. On the level of behaviour, the sub-system is *the inter-action system*, which is the organization of overt action among persons over time.

2. On the level of emotion, the sub-system is *group emotion*, which is the configuration of feelings among members and of their emotional responses to events that occur.

3. On the level of norms, the sub-system is the *normative system*, which is the organized, and largely shared, ideas about what members should do and feel, about how these should be regulated, and about what sanctions should be applied when behaviour does not coincide with the norms.

4. On the level of goals, the sub-system is *the technical system*, which is the set of ideas about what the group should accomplish, and the plans about how it is to be accomplished.

5. On the level of values, the sub-system is *the executive system*, which consists of interpretations of what the group *is*, the ideas about what would be desirable for it to become, and ideas about how it might so become.

The degree to which these five sub-systems are interrelated and the nature of such interrelationships in any particular group are matters for empirical research, and some findings will be discussed below.

Four developmental phases of group membership

Phase 1: Interaction and group emotion An interesting aspect of Mills's approach is that it enables one to imagine the experience of group membership as it develops over time. Mills presents a new-comer's progress into the group as a gradual four-phase process of participation. First, perhaps after some preliminary observation and attempts to make sense of what is going on, he begins to take part and to experience feelings toward the other members. For example, he answers a question put to him and feels slightly frightened by the tone of voice of one of the members. After a little while, he may start to like another member and ask a question himself. In effect, he has entered into the interaction sub-system and the group emotion.

A sequence of interaction—whether asking or answering questions, expressing agreement or disagreement, defending or attacking—quickly becomes ordered. In addition, the performance of particular kinds of acts tends to be differentially distributed among the group members. Some individuals will tend to initiate action while others mainly respond. Murray (1951), for example, has distinguished between proactions and reactions. Unless artificial restraints on inter-member communication are imposed, interaction in a spontaneously formed group will lead to the development of a hierarchy based on the type and frequency of contribution. This hierarchy basically reflects the unequal distribution of skill within a group faced with a particular task, and the consequent differentiation of proactivity can be related to the balance of power among group members (Richardson *et al.*, 1969). In fact, one of the most consistent findings in task-oriented groups is that the person who talks most and initiates interaction is seen by the other members as the group leader (Borgatta and Bales, 1956).

A person's part in the structured sequence of acts, according to Mills, is his *behavioural role*. Behavioural roles are usually inter-dependent in that a change in one results in an automatic change in another. When the newcomer in the above example stopped answering and began to ask questions, someone else would probably have to take on an 'answering' role.

In the same example, when the new member expresses his fear the member who first spoke in a harsh tone might feel dismay. If the former's fear were to diminish eventually the latter might experience relief. A person's part in a configuration of feelings, also mutually interdependent, is his *primordial role*. The total structure of primordial roles constitues the group emotion. In this context, Bion's basic assumption groups, Whitaker and Liebermann's focal conflict and Freud's primal horde are structures of group emotion. Mill's concept of group emotion includes the needs and drives that initially impel people to form groups; satisfactions and frustrations occasioned by experience in the group; interpersonal likes and dislikes within the group and feelings of attachment or alienation in relation to the group itself. The elements and processes that together comprise the group emotion may be conscious or unconscious, and they influence the range of action, thought, beliefs and expression of group members.

The concept of group emotion was developed by Redl, (1942; see also Ringwald, 1974) who attempted to supplement Freud's formulation (1921) that a primary psychological group was '*a number of individuals who have put one and the same object in the place of their ego ideal and have consequently identified themselves with one another in their ego*'. Redl accepted the validity of this formula, but he was able to extend it in the light of Freud's own subsequent development of the concepts of the super-ego and identification, on the one hand, and the differentiation of libido and aggression on the other.

Redl switched the focus from the 'leader' of a group to the various possible kinds of 'central' or 'focal' person around whom instinctual and emotional events revolved. Of particular interest were those emotional events that were basic to group formation, i.e. the source or reason for the group's existence. Redl had practical experience of children's groups and had carried out investigations of behavioural contagion and the processes of social influence in groups (Lippitt *et al.*, 1952; Polansky *et al.*, 1950). He was able to discern in these groups ten roles which a central person can perform to evoke group formation. These roles are defined in terms of the psychodynamic function that they fulfil for the potential group members. In addition to Freud's 'leader', who appeals to the narcissism of the members and is incorporated into their ego ideal, Redl mentions two other objects of identification: the 'patriarchal sovereign' whose conscience members incorporate into their own superego, and the 'tyrant', where the mechanism of identification is similar but is an identification with an aggressor out of fear rather than out of love. The '*love object*' and the 'object of aggressive drives' (i.e. the scapegoat) allow members basic instinctual gratification. The 'organiser', 'seducer', 'hero', 'bad influence' and 'good influence' are all relatively unconflicted personalities who, through the performance of 'initiatory acts', provide a service to the conflict-ridden egos of the members. This service can be either to permit the expression of libidinal or aggressive drives which would otherwise have been impossible because of guilt or anxiety, or to reinforce a defence or sublimation by affording a solution to the ego's conflict in the direction of moral values. The group conductor will easily recognise these and other primordial roles such as the 'sick one', 'therapist', 'favourite', 'victim', etc.

Phase 2: The normative system   The first phase of group membership, therefore, involves the member's participation in what is done and felt, and his assumption of behavioural and primordial roles. In Mills's second phase, a member enters into the *normative sub-system* and becomes aware that the real significance of any act or feeling is given by the meaning attributed to it by the group members. An act or feeling can have a variety of meanings, which depend on the particular person and specified circumstance in which the act or feeling occurs. For example, in a prison certain acts like 'grassing' are condemned no matter who commits them; but longer-serving inmates may be entitled to make demands of staff that would be forbidden to newcomers. Since norms are ideas about what should and should not be done, felt or expressed by a certain member in a specific situation, they must be sufficiently flexible to accommodate diverse persons, times and occasions. Norms may be codified or informal, explicit or implicit, conscious or unconscious, easily demonstrable or evident only when breached (Mills, 1962):

> group norms are a set of statements about feelings and behaviour. They are cognitive and moral statements which screen, evaluate, prescribe, and proscribe feelings and actions. As statements they are distinct from feelings and from behaviour. They exist in symbolic form in the mind, and are elements of group culture.

The normative sub-system includes more than norms. To assess a group's normative system it is necessary to consider in addition to norms:

(1)   the definitions of deviance (acts that violate the range of permissable behaviours or feelings);
(2)   the relative importance of different norms;
(3)   the relative seriousness of deviant acts;
(4)   the scope of application of the norms (when is the individual immune); and
(5)   the means by which norms, sanctions and boundaries can be changed.

'Altogether the normative system refers to how social control *should* be exercised in the group' (Mills, 1962).

A new member finds himself confronted with the normative system as a social fact which exists outside himself and constrains his freedom. His *normative role* is the totality of ideas that he has about what a person in his position in the group should do, feel and express in relation to other members and about how he should control himself and others to maintain the system. If a member comes to accept this role, he will be welcomed by the group and granted the privileges of membership. Jackson (1959) has demonstrated in a study of reference group processes that the allocation of prestige among group members is based on compliance with norms as well as contribution to group goals. Festinger, Schachter and Back (1950) have investigated the subtle pressures exerted on deviant group members and showed that these members were relatively rejected in terms of sociometric choices. Other studies have emphasised the positive functions that a deviant performs for the other group members. Dentler and Erikson (1959) suggested that the presence of a deviant helps other members to clarify and see the value of the group norms. Comparing themselves with the deviant, members can better understand how their normative behaviour is related and essential to the survival of the group as well as to the attainment of individual and collective goals. Feldman (1969) looked at the relationship between scapegoating and social rejection, on the one hand, and group integration, on the other. Although he did not find a significant relationship between intense scapegoating behaviour and either interpersonal or functional integration (a greater mutual liking among the other group members or a higher degree of complementary role specialisation and effectiveness), Feldman did discover both high and low correlations with normative integration (a consensus on group relevant behaviours). He concluded that scapegoating may sometimes serve the function of norm consensus. This may be particularly evident when there is no objective basis for members' beliefs except social validation (cf., for example, Festinger, 1950). Finally, Deutsch and Gerard (1955) pointed out that the early conformity experiments of Asch (1951, 1952) and Sherif (1936) did not distinguish between influence exerted by information purporting to be evidence about reality and normative social influence since the subjects were not actually taking part as group members. The fact that the mere presence of other people, who express judgements about reality, could have effects on an individual's own perception only hinted at the enormously powerful influence of group norms. This study found that even when normative influence was small group members were virtually unable to resist.

Phase 3: The technical system   The third phase of group membership is identification with the group goal, entry into the technical system, and the performance of an *instrumental role* (Mills, 1962). The concept of group goal refers to a desirable collective action. As a mental construct, the group goal exists in the minds of individual members, but it is not the sum of individual goals; its referent is the group as a whole. For example, a staff team in a psychiatric hospital is comprised of numerous individuals, each of whom will have his own goal—the satisfaction of needs to belong, the development of professional competence, or advancement in a career structure. The group goal, however, must be defined socially in terms of the institution's relationship to its external environment and to its clients (the patients). As such, goal-setting at a group level is a dynamic process which must take into account what the environment is willing to support and what it demands as well as the ideas of members themselves (cf. for example Thompson and McEwen, 1958). Without the successful accomplishment of the group goal—for a hospital this might be the recognition of its treatment programme effectiveness—individual goals may be unattainable.

The technical system consists of the co-ordinated 'know how', skills and techniques of the group; standards for evaluating the effectiveness of individual performances of assigned activities; and criteria for assessing the success or failure of the task as a whole. When a member performs an instrumental role within this system, he recognises, accepts and commits himself to the group goal. This implies that he gives the group goal ' . . . higher priority than his own goals, the group's norms, and the existing pattern of emotional relationships among members, including his own popularity and personal comfort' (Mills, 1962). The instrumental role is a member's specific assignment and the criteria he uses to guide and evaluate the effectiveness of his own and others' work performance.

An extensive research literature exists regarding the conditions that determine group task effectiveness and productivity. Some of the earliest social psychological investigations of 'social facilitation' were of the 'alone and together' type, and sought to establish when an individual working alone was less or more efficient than a group. (Hare, 1962, reviews the literature on task effectiveness.) Four studies are of particular relevance to Mills's analysis of instrumental roles and the technical system.

Guetzkow (1968) distinguished *role differentiation*, which is related to external and internal facts such as task characteristics, restriction of communications and the nature of the group goal, from the *effective interlocking of roles* into a structure. The actual organisation of instrumental roles depends on whether activities comprising the task can be assembled into functional positions; members perceive the development and differentiation of roles; specific organisational planning occurs; and the intellectual ability of the group is high.

Deutsch (1949) found that role inter-dependence could either facilitate or hinder the performance of group tasks according to the incentives offered to members. If emphasis was placed on co-operation—member x's action clearly helped member y to progress towards the group goal—members tended to be 'promotively interdependent' and were motivated, friendly and productive. On the contrary, in competitive groups—where member x's actions hindered member y's progress—a condition of 'contrient interdependence' was brought about and productivity was much lower.

Thomas (1957) found that even maximum facilitative interdependence, which was positively related to group cohesiveness, productivity and feelings of mutual responsibility, also led to a high level of tension. He explained this as the result of a conflict between the individual group member's desire to be responsible and the consequent stretching of his performance capacity to contribute to the group effort. Thomas suggested that an optimum degree of interdependence might be found so as not to produce excessive tension, which he hypothesised might eventually impede productivity.

Finally, Raven and Rietsema (1957) examined the relationship between goal clarity and group members' feelings of security. They found that clarity did not correlate either with members' self-evaluations or with their evaluation of the group. But when the group goal was clear and the path towards it was structured, members were more attracted to the task, could perceive the role structure more correctly, and were willing to accept more influence from others.

Phase 4: The executive system   As a member successively enters new roles, his previous roles are altered. The normative role changes how a member acts and expresses his feelings; the instrumental role may require that the behavioural, primordial or normative roles be temporarily suspended. The attainment of a group goal may even lead to new systems of interaction, emotions and norms, with corresponding rearrangements of roles on each level. The fourth and final phase of Mills's description—entry into the executive role—entails the greatest transformation of membership, for the incumbent of this role takes full responsibility for the group and for the development of its capabilities.

Mills lists four features of the executive role:

(1)   identification with the total group rather than with parts or sub-systems and an awareness of the group's history, potentials, requirements and choices;

(2)   intervention in response to momentary situations to influence what the group will become;

(3)   decommitment from all other role expectations; and

(4)   dual orientation to the group, seeing it simultaneously as an outsider and as a insider who is involved on all levels.

Since the executive role does not refer to a unique position in the group hierarchies but involves an approach to the situation and the performance of particular functions, it is potentially open to any member of the group. The executive system is, therefore, 'the set of all executive orientations and processes as they are distributed and organised among and performed by group members'. In essence, the executive system is the group's 'think-tank' where the function of assessment, reorganisation and the integration of experience are carried out (Mills, 1962).

The extent to which a group actually elaborates all five role systems discussed by Mills is a matter for empirical investigation. Theoretically, Mills believes that the purpose for which a group is formed will determine the minimum required elaboration. If a group meets for the purpose of immediate gratification, systems of interaction and group emotion are essential, for people must act and feel in order to be gratified. The normative system must be added to sustain the conditions of gratification over time. To pursue a collective goal demands a technical system of task functional roles. Finally, for purposes of self-determination and growth, an executive system is required. More complex orders of purpose entail more fully fledged role systems. Truncated groups, those with fewer role systems, are inherently limited in terms of attainable goals and minimise the role repertories available to individual members (Mills, 1962).

FIELD THEORY

The second theoretical approach to groups is rooted in Kurt Lewin's field theory and has been used by Cartwright and Zander in their anthology, *Group Dynamics Research and Theory* (1953, 1960, 1968).

The field

The concept of field is transposed from physics and also draws on the general insight of Gestalt psychology that the whole is different from the sum of its parts. The field is a totality of interdependent elements, all of which exert some force (having strength, direction and a point of application), which influences what a person does or does not do in any situation. As a concept, field is designed to reveal a 'cross-sectional view of the multiple causes of a bit of human behaviour' and to demonstrate the lawful relation between that behaviour and the momentary interplay of forces (Mills, 1962). Lewin (1936) stated his approach as follows:

One can apply a law only if one knows the nature of the concrete case with which one is dealing. Considered from this point of view the laws are nothing more than principles according to which the actual event may be derived from the dynamic factors of the concrete situation.

This relationship can be made clear by the following formulation: If one represents behaviour or any kind of mental event by B and the whole situation including the person by S, then B may be treated as a function of $S: B = f(S)$'.

The life space

Lewin developed his ideas in a number of writings, first in relation to individual psychology (1935, 1936; also see Deutsch, 1968a,b) where he conceived of the individual as located within and moving through a 'life space', 'the interaction between the person and the environment as it exists (has demonstrable effects) for him' (quoted in Durkin, 1964; cf. also Lewin, 1951). An expanded derivation of the above formula describes the whole situation (Lewin, 1936),

> by roughly distinguishing the person (P) and his environment (E). Every psychological event depends upon the state of the person and at the same time on the environment, although their relative importance is different in different cases. Thus we can state our formula $B = f(S)$ for every psychological event as $B = f(PE)$. . . . Every scientific psychology must take into account whole situations, i.e., the state of both person and environment. This implies that it is necessary to find methods of representing person and environment in common terms as parts of one situation. We have no expression in psychology that includes both. For the word situation is commonly used to mean environment . . . we shall use the term psychological life space to indicate the totality of facts which determine the behaviour of an individual at a certain moment.

The life space is a kind of personal field, a range of what is possible and not possible for a person at a specific time in a particular situation (Lewin, 1936):

> The different kinds of behaviour that occur in a certain situation are to be understood as belonging to a coherent system of 'possible' events that are in their totality an expression of the particular characteristics of the situation.
>
> The more we succeed in determining the details of the situation in this sense, the more the actual possibilities are limited. A complete determination of the life space would show which of the possibilities, given by its general structure, will be realised at the moment.

The themes that constantly reappear in this work are Lewin's emphasis on total situations, systematic rather than historical causation and dynamics.

The field theoretical definition of group

Subsequently, Lewin became interested in studying and effecting social change, and he applied his analysis to groups (1943, 1947a,

1948, 1951). A key series of articles from this period was included in the first issues of *Human Relations* (Lewin, 1947b,c) shortly before Lewin's death. (Incidentally, Bion's first paper on 'Experiences in Groups' appeared in the following number in 1948.) The first paper—'Frontiers in Group Dynamics: Concept, Method and Reality in Social Science; Social Equilibria and Social Change'—provided a concise exposition of Lewin's theory and experimental method, and it remains a unique example of group dynamics thinking. Lewin defined a group as a dynamic whole characterised by close interdependence of its members which may have specific structural properties that are similarly characterised by the relations between parts rather than by the parts or elements themselves.

This definition reflects the essence of the field theoretical approach in its emphasis on dynamic interdependent relations which occur at two levels of conceptualisation. On the first level, individuals engage in a continuous process of adaptation to one another's needs and mutual problems. As a consequence, their interpersonal behaviour becomes patterned—roles develop, sub-groups form, a division of labour emerges, differentiations of authority, power and status occur, norms and values are systematised, and a hierarchy of goals is established. On the second level, these social entities are themselves dynamically interrelated and make up the group-as-a-whole which is distinct from its parts.

The social field

Lewin then suggested that a group, analogous to an individual, will have a location within its environment, and he proposed the term 'social field' to denote the totality of co-existing psychological and social forces acting on the group (Lewin, 1951). Again, he stressed the underlying ideas of structure, ecological setting and basic possibilities for movement (locomotion) in the field. The scientific prediction of group behaviour depends on assessing the magnitudes and directions of the forces within the field and determining their distribution. Attention must be directed to the needs of group members, the structural properties of the group (goals, standards, values etc.), and to how the group views the situation relative to other groups. In functional terms, $Bg = f(PGE)$: group behaviour or a group event is a function of elements in the members' personalities, the group and the group's environment (cf. Mills, 1962). A social happening, like an individual action, occurs in and is a resultant of a totality of co-existing social entities, structured according to their relative position in the field.

Implicit in this theory is the proposition that observable, surface events are functions of many underlying dynamic variables. Instead of specifying linear relationships, explanation would ideally be in terms of circular, causal processes which interrelate configurations of variables. For example, one such explanatory 'map' (March and Simon, 1958) hypothesises that the frequency of interaction in a group varies with the perception of shared goals and the satisfaction of individual needs, while the extent of interaction, in its turn, influences identification with the group; the more members identify with the group, however, the more they perceive goals as shared and the more satisfied they are. Jackson's study (1959) of staff relations in a mental health clinic illustrates another circular process. By means of a subtle, constant communication of evaluative signs and cues, members were informed whether or not they were valued by others. The more valued a member felt, the more attracted he was to the group and the more he conformed and contributed. Conformity and contributions, finally, determined his position in the prestige structure, which was the origin of the pattern of evaluative signs.

The field and change

In a posthumously published second article—'Frontiers in Group Dynamics II: Channels of Group Life: Social Planning and Action Research' (1947c)—Lewin addressed himself to the problem of change. He saw a given state of events as a 'quasi-stationary equilibrium' maintained by the particular distribution of forces in the total social field. These forces will have opposed qualities, some tending to promote change (to move away from the equilibrium) and others tending to resist change (to maintain the equilibrium). Changes may be introduced either by adding forces in the desired direction or diminishing opposing forces, but excessive tensions within the field may be avoided by reducing the opposing forces. To be effective, any process of change involves three steps: (1) the unfreezing of the current equilibrium; (2) moving to a new level; and (3) freezing a new force field around the desired equilibrium. Since the field is characterised by interdependence, change in one part will have ramifications throughout.

A classic group dynamics experiment

An experimental investigation conducted by Lewin and his colleagues White and Lippitt (Lewin and Lippitt, 1938; Lewin *et al.*, 1939; Lippitt, 1939; White and Lippitt, 1960) illustrates the application of a field theoretical approach to the study of groups. Their research, carried out in 1939–40, was probably the most influential early project in the area of group dynamics; it exemplifies Lewin's dictum (1947c) that by 'doing something with groups' the reality of social entities could be established.

The object of study was what White and Lippitt (1960) called *social climate:*

> The primary aim of the first study was to develop techniques for creating and describing the 'social atmosphere' of children's clubs and for quantitatively recording the effects of varied social atmosphere upon group life and individual behaviour. Two degrees of control of group life, labelled 'democratic' and 'authoritarian' were used as the experimental variables, [quoted in Cartwright and Zander, 1968].

A second study added a *laissez-faire* condition. Four five-member groups of ten-year-old boys who met after school for hobby activities were used as subjects. The groups were roughly equivalent on a number of dimensions including sociometric characteristics, personality and intellectual, physical and socio-economic status. Four adults were trained to provide all three experimental treatments, and they were rotated between the clubs at six-week intervals. At each transition, the adults changed their behaviour so that each club experienced each treatment from every adult. All clubs met in the same setting, two at a time in adjacent spaces, with a common pool of equipment. The same activities were also used, by imposing on the 'authoritarian' groups those activities that were freely selected in 'democratic' groups; activities in the *'laissez-faire'* situation were basically similar.

In the *democratic* treatment, all policies were determined by group discussion and decision, encouraged and assisted by the adult leader. When technical advice was required in order to carry out a group task, the leader suggested at least two alternative procedures. Members could work with whomever they chose, and the division of labour was left to the group. Finally, the leader was objective (task-oriented) in his praise and criticism, and tried to be a regular group member without doing too much of the work himself.

The *authoritarian* treatment was characterised by complete policy determination by the adult leader, who dictated the activity steps one at a time; task clarity was, consequently, very low and it was difficult to anticipate successive steps. The leader also specified the work task and workmate of each member. Praise and criticism tended to be personal, and the leader remained detached from the group except when he was demonstrating a particular activity.

In the *laissez-faire* groups, leader participation was minimal. There was complete freedom for group or individual decision and, after supplying material and clarifying that he would advise if requested, the leader took no more part except infrequently to comment on the activities. No attempt to praise, criticise or regulate the course of events was made.

During each session, a quantitive account of social interaction, a minute-by-minute record of group structure, a qualitative interpretation of significant inter-member transactions and a continuous script of all conversations were made by four observers. At regular intervals, several test events took place: the leader arrived late; the leader left for an indeterminate time; a stranger arrived and in the leader's absence criticised the work of an individual member or of the group.

The more important results of this research concern the effects of the different treatments on the boys' behaviour towards the adult and towards each other. *Laissez-faire* groups were not the same as 'democratic' groups in several respects: (1) less work was accomplished in the former and it was of lower quality; (2) more play took place in the *laissez-faire* groups (a similar result has been found in leaderless psychotherapy groups, according to Bednar and Lawlis, 1971). The boys preferred 'democratic' groups, according to interviews. Although the quantity of work done in 'authoritarian' groups was somewhat larger, work motivation and originality were greater in 'democratic' conditions. The most discontent was expressed in 'authoritarian' groups, but members reacted to their discontent in two ways. They either showed a great deal of hostility and aggression, often directed at scapegoats (the stranger or the other group); or they responded submissively and apathetically, relied dependently on the leader, and demonstrated almost no capacity for initiating action. In 'democratic' treatments, there was more group-mindedness (mutual praise, sharing property, spontaneous sub-group formation), friendliness and satisfaction with the club activities.

Lewin (1947b) assessed these data on the levels of aggression in line with his concept of quasi-stationary equilibria. The level of perpetrated aggression is understood either in terms of an increase in the strength of forces towards more aggression (such as harsh criticism or rough games) or a decrease in forces tending towards less aggression (fewer friendships among members, absence of adult leader, diminished 'we feeling'). When a member was transferred from a 'democratic' to an 'authoritarian' group, or vice versa, the new member showed the level of dominance reached by the other members of that group before the change; this demonstrates an equilibrium-maintaining force field within the group. Likewise, the amount of aggression received, the passive property of being attacked (scapegoating) is seen in terms of the forces characteristic of the group, the particular individual and his relàtion to his surroundings, i.e. the aggressiveness of members, the social atmosphere, the extent to which the member provokes or invites attack or fights back.

In another example based on the Western Electric studies, Lewin suggested that the forces impinging on a work group's productivity would include such things as the strain of hard or fast work, the system of incentives and rewards, the sub-culture (norms) of the group, the desire to be 'average', and the fear that increased efficiency might lead to pressure from the foreman to maintain the new level.

'Group-carried' change

For the group therapist, who is vitally concerned with promoting change in the personalities of his patients and in the circumstances of his group, one of the great merits of Lewin's work is precisely its illumination of the complexities entailed in any process of change. Lewin's analysis of the *status quo* as an equilibrium held in place by a configuration of forces highlights the power of targeting change at the group rather than at the individual, especially when beliefs, conduct or attitudes are demonstrably anchored in a group. For successful efforts to change the individual alone may lead to his estrangement from his group or to group pressure with consequent effects on his self-concept and self-esteem. Lewin proposed a theorem to the effect that the greater the social value of a group standard, the greater will be an individual's resistance to move away. Changes that are 'group-carried' involve a perception by the individuals concerned that their group is prepared to sanction an alteration of its standard. The change has a social value, which limits resistance due to the relation between the individual and the group. In the group change process, discussion would promote unfreezing of the current equilibrium (the individuals' dependence on a valued standard), proposals of alternatives would lead the group to a new level, and a decision would freeze a new force field around the new equilibrium. The forces inherent in a decision include an individual's wish to be seen to stick to his decision and his genuine commitment to the group (Lewin, 1947c).

The 'gate-keeper' as change agent

During World War II, because of the difficulties in obtaining certain customary foods, Lewin was engaged by the US Government in a study to find out how best to change people's eating habits; and he focused his analysis on the channels through which food passed before it was actually served at the table (Lewin 1943, 1947c). On the one hand, there was the field comprised of market forces which determined how a particular food was produced, wholesaled, distributed, displayed on a shop shelf, and finally purchased. On the other hand, there was the domestic force field comprised of the tastes, preferences, and eating habits of particular households and families. A *gate region* is a location between two such constellations of decisively different forces, and the fate of a unit (food) in the whole channel depends on what happens at the gate. Gate regions are governed by rules or by 'gate-keepers', who may be individuals or groups. In this case Lewin found that an individual, the housewife, had a decisive influence on which foods moved through the channel and were eventually consumed.

In psychotherapy groups the therapist occupies simultaneously a number of such gate regions. From a psychoanalytic point of view, he stands at the intersections between the fields of inter-nalised object relations, psychic structures (ie, ego, super-ego), the total personality, the group, and the social organisation (or environment) of which the group is a part (Kernberg, 1975). From a sociological perspective, the group leader who performs Mills's

(1962) executive role is a 'gate-keeper' between the internal role systems of the group as well as between the existing group and its potential.

Turquet (1974a) elaborates the Tavistock conception of leadership (Rice, 1963, 1965) as a boundary function. The leader occupies the interface between the group system and its environment, and he must consistently define and maintain the primary task of the group in relation to the environment. This requires simultaneous participation in and observation of the group.

Whitaker and Liebermann (1965) describe the leader as experiencing the affects comprising the group focal conflict without actually participating in its generation or expression; he is at once in touch with and outside of the group.

Cartwright and Zander's application of field theory

Cohesiveness and group pressures

For Cartwright and Zander (1953, 1960, 1968), following Lewin, the group is a kind of force field, characterised by interdependence among its constituent units (individuals). Forces may tend to attract a person to the group; to induce him to involve himself more intimately, or to leave; or to resist and repel attempts to join. For example, in lower status positions forces act to restrain the upward communication of critical comments (Kelley, 1951) and to encourage irrelevant or submissive communications which serve to reduce the threat inherent in an asymmetrical power relationship (Hurwitz *et al.*, 1968). By reinforcing approved and punishing disapproved behaviour, group interaction draws the more valued members into central positions and excludes those who do not contribute (Jackson, 1959). The *'cohesiveness'* of a group is the constellation of such forces at any one time, a resultant of all forces acting on members to stay in the group which takes into account the attractiveness of alternative memberships (cf. also Festinger *et al.*, 1950). Membership is a boundary that, once crossed, will have a number of consequences.

One of the most important consequences of membership is that a person experiences pressures to conform to the beliefs, values and standards (even to the definitions of reality) of the group. The extent to which a member accepts group pressures to uniformity will depend on the attractiveness of membership to him and on the power of the group over its members, which is related to the group's cohesiveness. In effect, the power (P) of a group is only equal to the strength of forces on a member to remain in the group(S): $P = S$. If the group tries to induce a larger change than force S, the member will leave the group (Schachter *et al.*, 1951). These interrelationships actually describe another circular process which Cartwright (1968) has analysed in detail. Group cohesiveness varies with (1) the *incentive properties* of the group (attractiveness of or similarities between members, the attractiveness of group goals, activities, the nature of its leadership, atmosphere or prestige); (2) the *motivations of members* (needs for affiliation, friendship, rewards, recognition); (3) their *expectancies* concerning outcome (a subjective estimate of the probability that membership will insure the realisation of goals or the satisfaction of needs); and (4) the *comparison* level (a general conception of what outcomes group membership should provide on the basis of other group experience). In turn, the more cohesive a group, the more it can (1) hold its members; (2) exert power over them; (3) count on their participation and loyalty; (4) affect their feelings of personal security; and (5) influence their self-evaluations (cf. also Pepitone and Reichling, 1955; Back, 1951; Festinger, 1950; Schachter *et al.*, 1951; Festinger *et al.*, 1950).

Power

An analysis of the determinants and consequences of power and influence assumes a position of particular importance for understanding the nature of group pressures. Cartwright and Zander (1968), Cartwright (1959, 1965); and French and Raven (1959) distinguish between several resources or bases of power (the capacity to influence others), among which they include *reward power, coercive power, legitimate power, expert power* and *referent power* (based on identification or a desire to be like an admired person). If O is the agent exerting influence and P the one influenced, the range of O's power over P depends on the base of O's power. Legitimate power, grounded in a position of authority, will probably be more acceptable than coercive power; the power to reward may effectively influence overt behaviour, but referent power may influence beliefs and feelings as well. As the study by Lewin, Lippitt and White showed, the possession or non-possession of power affects the actions and feelings of group members, and groups will differ as to the bases of power allowed to members and the distribution of power within the group. For example, in therapeutic communities where the values of role-blurring and egalitarian democracy are strongly held, doctors are expected by other staff members to surrender their legitimate power which is derived from a formal position in the medical hierarchy. Their expert power is also occasionally depreciated, particularly when it rests on a medical model of emotional disturbance. An important implication of Cartwright and Zander's work is that a group power structure must be conceptually differentiated and related to the five system levels discussed by Mills.

Goals

The field theoretical conception of the group located in an environment (social field) underlies Cartwright and Zander's (1968) definition of the group goal:

> Whenever it is possible to assert that some location is relatively preferred for a group and that a sequence of efforts to change the group's location will terminate when it is reached, we will designate that location as the group's goal. If a group changes its location, we will speak of group locomotion. For group locomotion to occur it is usually necessary for the group to perform a sequence of group actions; a sequence that leads to a preferred location may be thought of as a path through the group's environment to its goal.

The group's goals, like other forces within the group, can act as an inducing vector; once established, group members are expected to work towards its realisation, but acceptance of any particular group goal will vary among individuals to the extent that they are attracted to membership. Commitment varies with cohesiveness and compliance. The rules and procedures for combining individual preferences for a group's location in its social field constitute the decision-making process. Participation in this process is differentially distributed among group members and is associated with the distribution of power. A member who feels that he is an effective participant in goal-setting is likely to be more highly motivated to contribute his effort and skill than one who is not consulted (Coch and French, 1948).

The arrangement for distributing rewards will also affect motivation. If, for example, each member's reward is independent of both total group output and his own contribution (fixed in advance), little incentive to increase either output would be expected. On the other hand, if rewards are contingent on both group and individual achievements, contributions to both are encouraged. However, the latter arrangement produces a complicated dilemma, for while each member would want others to contribute to the group goal, he would not want any other's efforts to exceed his own (Cartwright and Zander, 1968; see also Thomas, 1957). Deutsch (1949) suggested that 'the communication of ideas, co-ordination of efforts, friendliness, and pride in one's group which are basic to group harmony and effectiveness appear to be disrupted when members see themselves to be competing for mutually exclusive goals' (quoted in Cartwright and Zander, 1968).

Groups are vitally affected by whether they succeed in attaining their goals. Success may lead to greater group cohesiveness, higher aspirations and greater self-confidence on the part of members, who will in turn be more committed and more willing to accept influence attempts. Cohesiveness can increase a group's capacity to deal with threats or obstacles to goal attainment (Pepitone and Reichling, 1955). It is clear, however, that group productivity is not automatically increased as the group's power to induce compliance grows. Cohesiveness does affect productivity, but the direction depends on the norms of the group. In some circumstances, relatively low-cohesive, low-power groups might be more productive than a successful, high-power one which could use power to freeze productivity at a certain level. In other cases, a cohesive group will not necessarily use its power; i.e., there may not be norms for some activities and behaviours (Festinger *et al.*, 1950). Group failure to achieve objectives, on the other hand, may have the opposite effects, for a decline in cohesiveness may make future goal attainment even less probable.

Leadership

An act of leadership is one that either helps to maintain and strengthen the group or facilitates the group's movement towards its preferred location in its social field. Leadership is, therefore, defined functionally in relation to goals. The two basic leadership functions are initiating task structure and preserving the social–emotional solidarity of the group, and frequently the leadership contributions of an individual will tend to be more concentrated in one or the other of these areas. Style and personality both influence the degree to which the performance of leadership functions will be effective. For example, and as a minimum, a member must know the requirements for attaining the goal, and he must feel capable of carrying out the necessary actions. Korten (1962) found that authoritarian leaders were preferred when group goals assumed greater importance than individual goals and when there were ambiguities which obscured the path to attaining the group goals. When ambiguities did not create distress and the realisation of group goals was not seen as a prerequisite to the attainment of individual goals, more democratic leadership was sought. Summarising a fifteen-year programme of research comprising thirty-five studies of 1,600 groups, Fiedler (1968) remarked that the effectiveness of a group depends on the fit between leadership style and the specific situation, particularly the group task situation. In accordance with the field theoretical perspective, Cartwright and Zander emphasise the situational determinants of leadership such as the expectations of group members and the goal structure of the group. Although leadership is not equally distributed within the group, it is potentially open to all members (cf. also the discussion of Mills's executive role).

INTERACTION PROCESSES

Homans (1951, 1961, 1968) has suggested that much small group research is really the study of elementary social behaviour, of the face-to-face interaction that comprises only part of the total behaviour of groups as units. In fact, Homans defined a group in terms of quantities of interaction (1951):

> If we say that individuals A, B, C, D, E . . . form a group, this will mean that at least the following circumstances hold. Within a period of time, A interacts more with B, C, D, E, . . . than he does with M, N, L, O, P, . . . whom we choose to consider outsiders or members of other groups. B also interacts more often with A, C, D, E, . . . than he does with others, and so on for the other members of the group. It is possible just by counting interactions to map out a group quantitively distinct from others.

It is clear that, from the systems and field theoretical perspectives, groups develop internal differentiations with respect to roles, power, status, etc. These differentiations structure the interactions that occur within the group; that is, they shape, facilitate, restrain and delimit the possible actions available to members. However, the *process of interaction* itself—the quantity, sequence and inter-relation of acts over time—has attracted the attention of group researchers as much as the structure that subsequently emerges from it. Structure and process are complementary concepts. The third orientation within group dynamics employs a model for the analysis of interaction processes which permits a sequential classification of acts.

The classification of acts: content

An example is the work of Hare (1962). At the highest level of generality, Hare believes that human behaviour is concerned primarily with problem solving, starting with the problem of survival. Human behaviour in groups will also be directed towards solutions to the members' various problems as well as to the problems inherent in maintaining the functioning of the group itself. Therefore, in any group, two levels of problem may be distinguished: *individual problems* and *group problems*. On each level, a problem will have one of two basic contents; problems will be related to *tasks*, or to *social–emotional issues*. At the group level the task is to solve the publicly stated problem of the group, to achieve the primary purpose for which the group was formed. Social–emotional problems are those arising from the need to establish an interpersonal structure or 'pecking order' such as when dealing with shared anxieties, competition, and intimacies between the members. On the individual level, the task is the individual's publicly stated goal or reason for joining the group. Social–emotional problems include his efforts to cope with membership and with the problem of self-integration (intra-psychic strains).

Regardless of level, any act may be classified according to its problem content. An act or contribution may be conscious or unconscious, verbal or non-verbal, ranging from a posture, gesture, expression of feeling, word, or phase to a complete sentence or longer intervention, depending on the object of investigation. In the area of task behaviour, the minimum number of categories would include observing, hypothesising and formulating action.

69

In the area of social–emotional behaviour the minimum number of categories would include control and affection. (Incidentally, although the emphasis here is on process, this type of category system may also be used to describe the structure of interaction; i.e., expectations for behaviour could be primarily in the category of observing for new members of a group; in a family, the father may perform the role of task leader and the mother that of social–emotional leader, or vice-versa.)

The classification of acts: form

Process analysis also involves an examination of the form of interaction. By form, Hare (1962) refers to the *communication network* and the *rate of interaction*. The communication network of a group is composed of the channels of regularised message flow between members (Burges, 1969). A complete description of interaction would record the extent to which each available channel is actually open for input and output, i.e. the extent to which each member uses his channels (output) and how others respond (input). The correlation between output and input is usually high; those who speak most are spoken to most often (Bales *et al.* 1951). The interaction rate or frequency is operationally defined variously by the number of acts, the ratio of number to duration of acts, or the number multiplied by the average duration of acts.

Communication

Bavelas (1950) mentions the general relation between communication, control and authority and has studied how communication patterns affect the group's work, leadership, organisation and resistance to disruption. He introduced the notion of 'distance' in a communication net which is defined as the sum of the number of links all members must go through to communicate with everyone else. The 'relative centrality' of a position X within the net is the distance divided by the sum of distances for position X. Bavelas found that the individual occupying the most central position tends to be seen as the leader. Occupancy of the more peripheral positions tends to be associated with lower morale. In high-centrality nets (for example where four peripheral members each can communicate only with a fifth), organisation develops more rapidly, is more stable and fewer errors occur, but morale is low.

The communication network may also affect the utilisation of insight, and when severe restraints are imposed a group task solution is hindered.

Burges (1969) has reviewed the major communications research projects from 1951 to 1964 and found that the reported differences in problem-solving effectiveness between a relatively low-distance net (the wheel) and a relatively high-distance net (the circle) tended to level off if incentives (reinforcement of correct answers) and a transition period from acquisition to steady state of solution rate were provided. He concluded that perhaps 'several kinds of social structures can be equally efficient in producing desired ends *if* under certain structures the members receive reinforcements of greater amounts, at more frequent intervals, or at higher probabilities' (Burges, 1969).

Category systems

Hare's category system for classifying acts is related to his theory of groups as problem-solving units, and the derivation of particular category systems for process analysis has depended on the theoretical position of the observer. Chapple (1942) categorised all acts of clients in structured business or psychiatric interview into action or silence. Piaget (1926), studying the functions of language, categorised typical interaction patterns between children into eight categories: repetition, monologue, collective monologue, adapted information, criticism and derision, orders and threats, question, and answer. Moreno (1923) used notations for 'spontaneity states' and an 'action diagram' to describe action process in his theatre of spontaneity, the precursor of sociodrama and psychodrama. Ruesch and Prestwood (1950) have elaborated over 100 types of action categories to analyse process in therapy and counselling.

Interaction process analysis

By far the most influential category system has been developed by Bales (1950a,b, 1970); indeed, Hare's system essentially follows Bales's approach. Bales taught at one of the first small group seminars in 1946, and his laboratory for the study of small groups in the Department of Social Relations at Harvard University has become a major centre for group dynamics research (cf. Gibbard *et al.*, 1974). A close collaborator of Parsons, Bales shares the systems theory view that the small face-to-face group is an example of a social system. As such, the group elaborates means to deal with internal and external problems that arise out of the process of interaction among the group members, on the one hand, and between the group and its environment, on the other. The group's structural features are emergent solutions to various issues which are posed by the context of interaction. For example (Bales, 1950a):

> It is to the advantage of every individual in a group to stabilize the potential activity of others toward him, favorably if possible, but in any case in such a way that he can predict it. Structure thus partially solves the problems of interaction which might result from inter-personal conflict [quoted in Durkin, 1964].

To solve problems and make decisions, group members must with reasonable efficiency be able to communicate and to exchange information in order to define the situation that confronts them. They must evaluate that situation and work out a common attitude towards it. Finally, they must make a decision from among alternative courses of action; i.e., they must exercise control over competing proposals. In addition to the three basic *instrumental functions* of communication, evaluation and control, problem-solving requires that members indicate whether they accept or reject the direction in which the group is moving, that they cope with tensions, and that the group itself holds together. The latter *social–emotional functions* are dynamically related to the instrumental functions. Bales's work has demonstrated how attempts to reach a task solution tend to disrupt the solidarity of the group. When consequent attempts are made to integrate the group, task efficiency diminishes, for involvement in social–emotional activity leaves less time and energy for work. Bales (1953) called the cyclical swing between efforts to complete the task and attempts to hold the group together (and satisfy members' needs) the equilibrium problem.

Bales's category system is closely related to his theoretical position. He focused exclusively on the problem-solving relevance of overt behaviour in groups. In his original formulation, Bales was not concerned with the substantive content of statements (ideas or emotions), the intent of the actor, or feelings and thoughts aroused in the course of action. Subsequently, however, he extended his analysis to attitude and value statements, the interpretation of group fantasy themes, and to the interpersonal perception of group members after meetings. Bales described his method as follows (1970):

> The method of simultaneously classifying the quality of the act, who performs it, in relation to whom . . . is called *Interaction Process Analysis.* . . . The interaction categories do not classify *what* is said, that is, the content of the message, but rather *how* the persons communicate, that is, *who does what to whom in the process (time order)* of their interaction.
>
> People often do not pay much attention to the form of their interaction, or do not have much control over it. They are usually more attentive to the content of what they are saying. But they unintentionally convey much in their manner, and this is intuitively understood by most of their listeners. A language of manner, or form of interaction, in fact exists along with the more explicit language, and is regularly employed in interpersonal communication, but at a low level of awareness by some, and with quite imperfect understanding. Although the basic sequences are easy to grasp, the quantitative balances and relations of rates to each other are quite subtle, and soon reach a level of complication beyond easy conscious control. This is especially true when one takes into account the nature of activity *received* by the individual as well as the nature of what he initiates.

Interaction process-categories

Bales (1950b) uses twelve categories to collect process data. He divides the social–emotional area into *positive reactions* ('green-light') and *negative reactions* ('red-light') to ongoing task activity. The positive reactions are: *Category 1*—shows solidarity; raises other's status; gives help and reward. *Category 2*—shows tension release; jokes, laughs and shows satisfaction. *Category 3*—agrees, showing passive acceptance; understands, concurs and complies. The negative social–emotional reactions include: *Category 10*—disagrees, showing passive rejection and formality; withholds help. *Category 11*—shows tension and asks for help; withdraws out of field. *Category 12*—shows antagonism, deflating others' status and defending or asserting self.

The instrumental or task area is similarly divided into two sections, *attempted answers and questions*. Attempted answers include: *Category 4*—gives suggestion and direction, implying autonomy for others. *Category 5*—gives opinion, evaluation and analysis; expresses feelings and wishes. *Category 6*—gives orientation and information; repeats, clarifies and confirms. Questions are: *Category 7*—asks for orientation, information, repetition and confirmation. *Category 8*—asks for opinion, evaluation, analysis and expression of feeling. *Category 9*—asks for suggestion, direction and possible ways of action.

According to the classification, categories can be paired. Instrumental acts relevant to problems of communication (orientation) are scored in categories 6 or 7; those relevant to problems of evaluation in 5 or 8; those relevant to problems of control in 4 or 9. Social–emotional acts relevant to problems of decision are scored in categories 3 or 10; those relevant to problems of tension management in 2 or 11; and those relevant to problems of integration in 1 or 12. The observer scores all acts by determining the most appropriate category and indicates the frequency of acts as well as the actor and the receiver.

The equilibrium problem

One of Bales's findings, the equilibrium problem, has already been mentioned: 'The problem of equilibrium is essentially the problem of establishing arrangements . . . whereby the system goes through a repetitive cycle, within which all of the disturbances created in one phase are reduced in some other' (Bales, in Hare *et al.*, 1955). All groups must deal with the incessant swings between commitment to tasks and commitment to social–emotional requirements. Attempts to solve the group's task lead to the differentiation of roles of the members as to functions and gross amounts of participation. Sometimes a division of labour occurs in which one active member forces the task pace while another concerns himself with keeping the group together (Bales and Slater, 1955). Actors also tend to distribute their responses to others according to the latter's output (Bales *et al.*, 1951). Both types of differentiation may have status implications that threaten the existing balance of relations among the members and may, therefore, disturb the group's solidarity.

Phase movement

Bales also found what he called 'phase movement': 'Changes in quality of activity as groups move through time in order to solve their problems may be called phase problems' (Bales, in Hare *et al.*, 1955; Bales and Strodtbeck, 1951). If a group meeting was divided into three equal time-periods the predominant type of activity tended to shift from *communication* and *information-collecting* (in period 1) to *evaluation of information* (in period 2) to *control and decision-making* (in period 3). These phase movements in the group's progress towards a decision were correlated with a series of changes in the social–emotional area. Impairment of the group's solidarity increased as the emphasis passed from orientation to evaluation to control; there was a positive relation between the degree of control (pressing for a decision) and negative reactions. Once a decision had been reached, the 'red light' responses decreased and were replaced by positive social–emotional reactions (Bales and Strodtbeck, 1951).

In addition to his study of within-meeting phase movements, Bales looked at meeting-to-meeting trends in initially leaderless groups and identified several patterns of interaction. In a series of four meetings, positive social–emotional behaviour continually increased. Negative reactions peaked in the second meeting when a hierarchy was established; Bales referred to this peak as the 'status struggle' (Heinicke and Bales, 1955). When status consensus was high, task activity dropped. The tendency for groups to shift from a task to a friendship basis was so marked that many groups remained together long after completing their tasks (Turquet, 1974a, also remarks on this and considers it a characteristic of basic assumption groups). Groups that did not successfully negotiate the 'status struggle' had to spend more time sorting out social–emotional problems and tended to be less efficient; members were also less satisfied with the group experience. Finally, if members took part in a series of groups, each with different members, the 'status struggle' never occurred, and most efforts were of necessity directed toward getting to know the other members. No development could take place and each group of the series was in effect meeting for the first time.

Interaction process analysis in clinical settings

Talland (1955) has used a slightly modified version of Bales's category system to study psychotherapy groups conducted at the

75

Maudsley Hospital by psychiatrists along group-analytic lines. Based on data from the first eight sessions, he found that there was no consistent phase movement from orientation to evaluation to control and attributed this result to the purpose of psychotherapy groups. Disturbances need to be held at a certain level. For example, if anxieties are constantly resolved, little work would be possible. Also, Talland pointed out that the discovery of problems rather than the solution, and the value of spontaneous emotional involvement rather than task discipline, temper the need for problem-solving (control) to rise at the end of every meeting. Psathas (1960a,b), using the complete set of categories including therapist-initiated acts, and sampling from beginning, middle and late periods of the sessions, substantiated Talland's finding that phase movements within single sessions did not clearly develop. But he did find support for such movements across all the sessions and also for the existence of equilibrium tendencies. Lennard and Bernstein (1960), Dunphy (1968), Blake (1953), Munzer and Greenwald (1957) and Roberts and Strodtbeck (1953) have also applied Bales's method to the study of interaction process in clinical settings.

Category systems for psychotherapy groups

Largely inspired by Bales's example, a number of researchers have developed category systems that are particularly relevant to the study of phase movements and trends in psychotherapy groups. Thelen (1954, Thelen et al., 1954; Stock and Thelen, 1958) converted Bion's notions of work and basic assumption groups into categories for the description of group processes. Behavioural classifications were derived from empirical data based on problem-solving experiments in which two levels of functioning, 'work' and 'emotionality', were noted. Four classes of 'emotionality'— (1) dependency on the leader, (2) fight, (3) flight (Thelen separated Bion's unified fight/flight assumption) and (4) pairing among the members, and four corresponding classes of 'work'—ranging from very little help to contributions that integrate the group activity with wider goals—were proposed. Each act is scored simultaneously on level of 'work' and 'emotionality'.

Hill and his colleagues (Hill, 1961; Martin and Hill, 1957) used a category system which modified Thelen's model. The Hill Interaction Matrix classifies activity into two dimensions, *content* and *work*. Contributions are categorised by content according to whether the general topic referred to is the group, something personal, or something concerning relationships. Work categories include responsive, conventional, assertive, speculative and confrontive. Groups move through phases of *orientation, exploration* and *production*.

Bennis and Shepard (1956) hypothesised that the principal obstacles to valid communication are found in the *orientations towards authority* (authority relations) and *intimacy* (personal relations) that members bring to the group. Classification is based on two areas of internal uncertainty: dependency (how members relate to authority) and interdependence (how members relate to peers). 'Dependence and interdependence—power and love, authority and intimacy—are regarded as the central problems of group life' (Bennis and Shepard, in Gibbard *et al.*, 1974). Groups move regularly from preoccupation with authority to preoccupation with interpersonal relations. In the first, authority, phase, members negotiate successive problems of submissiveness and rebellion and move to a resolution in independence. In the second peer phase the movement is from identification to self-identity and to resolution in interdependence.

Theories of group development

It is clear from the examples cited that the development of category systems has led to comprehensive theories of group development. Bennis and Shepard conceptualise a cyclical, developmental process in which the sub-phases and resolution of authority problems overlap with the corresponding sub-phases and resolution of intimacy problems. This is probably close to Bion's own understanding of how combinations of work and basic assumption groups recurrently emerge.

Schutz (1958) distinguishes three fundamental dimensions of interpersonal behaviour based on human needs for *inclusion, control* and *affection*. Group interaction in any period of time is predominantly related to one of these needs. The developmental sequence of a group moves from emphasis on problems of inclusion to problems of control and finally to problems of affection, a cycle that may recur many times in the group's life. Problems of inclusion also predominate when a member is preparing to leave

77

the group or when the group itself is about to disband; in effect, the pattern is reversed: affection–control–inclusion.

Mann (1966; Mann *et al.*, 1967) formulated a conceptual framework of group development which passes through phases of concern with problems of *nurturance* (dependent stage), *control* (struggle with the leader), *sexuality* (inter-member relations) and *competence* (mature work). He also used a member–leader scoring system which focused on members' expressions of hostility and affection, showing dominance, counter-dominance and independence, expressions and denials of anxiety and depression, and expressions of self-esteem.

Slater's thesis (1966) is that many of the issues that societies and groups have faced in the past are re-enacted as new groups form and develop. Members must cope with anxieties over their lack of differentiation from each other and with frustration in their relationships with the leader. This is followed by an attack on the leader in order to incorporate his power and learning. Finally, there is a period of high morale and egalitarianism. Before the revolt, three entities were bound up together—the person of the leader, the group deity (object of dependency needs) and a set of abstract skills, qualities and powers desired by all members. Group development depends on separating these entities (in fantasy and through learning) so that skills become available to the members. To reach the point of revolt, the group passes through three phases. A phase of *generalised inhibition of hostile feelings* towards the leader with some displacement towards peers leads to a virtually total *direction of aggression towards the leader* as the revolt develops. After the revolt, *a taboo on inter-member conflict* is instituted, which is gradually relaxed. Slater's model echoes Freud's theories of the primal horde and the Oedipus conflict.

Finally, Tuckman (1965) has presented one of the most inclusive theories of group development. His review of the literature on developmental sequences in small groups, covering studies of therapy groups, T-groups, natural and laboratory groups, extracted the stages of development identified in those studies which Tuckman then synthesised in his own theory.

The contention is that any group, regardless of setting, must address itself to the successful completion of a task. At the same time, and often through the same behaviours, group members will be relating to one another interpersonally. The pattern of *interpersonal relationships* is referred to as *group structure* and is interpreted as the interpersonal configuration and interpersonal behaviours of the group at a point in time, that is, the way the members act and relate to one another as persons. The proposed distinction between the group as a social entity and the group as a task entity is similar to the distinction between the task-oriented functions of groups and the social–emtional–integrative functions of groups, both of which occur as simultaneous aspects of group functioning.

Tuckman (1965) discerns four stages of group development: in the social realm, the stages are *testing-dependence, conflict, cohesion* and *functional roles*. In the task realm, the sequence is *orientation, emotionality, relevant opinion exchange,* and the *emergence of solutions*.

Testing and dependence refer to activity that seeks to establish what interpersonal behaviours are acceptable in the group, based on the reactions of the therapist, trainer, leader or other members. The aim is to test the boundaries of the situation. Also, members relate to a central person or powerful group member, or to the existing norms or structures, in a dependent way, looking for guidance and support in the new situation. On the task level, members attempt to orient themselves, to identify the task and to find out how group experience will be useful. They will ask questions about the type of information needed and how to get it, and will basically evolve the 'ground rules' of the task.

At the second social level, *intra-group conflict*, the most outstanding feature is lack of unity. Hostility is directed towards the leader or other members as a means of expressing individuality and resisting the formation of group structure. This period is characterised by uneven interaction, infighting, polarisation and the conflict between progression into interpersonal relationships and regression to dependent security. On the task level, members express emotional resistance to the demands of the work. They respond to the discrepancy between personal motivation and that required by the task.

Stage three at the social level comprises *the development of group cohesion*. Members accept the group and one another, generate new norms to maintain solidarity and facilitate mutual relationships, and tend to avoid overt conflicts. Harmony is the ultimate value. On the task level there is a wide-ranging exchange of relevant information and maximum acceptance of influence. Members reveal themselves and discuss other group members openly.

Finally, the fourth stage at the social level is *functional role relatedness*. The subjective relationships between the members have been worked out, and members can now perform roles that enhance task activities. Role structure is no longer an issue and does not present an obstacle to task efficiency. On the task level, solutions emerge and energy previously invested in the structural realm can be devoted to the constructive application of insights.

In some groups this four-stage developmental sequence may be preceded by a pre-stage in which there is resistance, silence and hostility. Members must be won over and their isolation or un-shared behaviour overcome. A new patient's group in the therapeutic community or pre-therapy role induction and socialisation may fulfil this function.

The theory may be encapsulated in four terms:

(1) *forming* (orientation, testing and dependence);
(2) *storming* (resistance to group influence and task);
(3) *norming* (in-group, intimate discussion with new standards and roles; and
(4) *performing* (interpersonal structure as a tool for task activities).

Tuckman's discussion of the application of this theory to psychotherapy groups will be an appropriate conclusion to a chapter on group dynamics, for it demonstrates how a wider view of groups can illuminate and guide clinical practice.

Many therapists have described the opening stage of testing–dependence. Bion's basic assumption *dependency group* is the prototype for this first phase. Bach (1954) noted the initial situation testing and leader dependence. Mann and Semrad (1948) emphasised how the group tests the tolerance limits of both leader and members. Corsini (1957) wrote of the initial hesitant participation of the members, characterised variously as a period of orientation, information, and testing (Grotjahn, 1950; Powdermaker and Frank, 1948), acclimatisation (King, 1959) and attachment to the group (Schindler, 1958). On the task level, the descriptions usually include references to indirect attempts to discover the nature and boundaries of the task (Bion, 1961) involving the discussion of irrelevant and partially relevant issues (Martin and Hill, 1957) peripheral problems, immediate behaviour problems, symptoms

(Bach, 1954), criticisms of the institutional environment (Mann and Semrad, 1948) and intellectualisation. Also, there are attempts at orientation to the task. Members search for the meaning of therapy, define the situation, try to establish a relationship with the therapist, exchange information (Grotjahn, 1950) and express suspiciousness and fear (Corsini, 1957).

In stage two, the structure is characterised by intra-group conflict, defensiveness, competition and jealousy. Bion's fight/flight implies conflict or attempts to withdraw. Other accounts mention a crisis period with arguments, broken rules and structural collapse (Parker, 1958); sharp fluctuations of relationship (Powdermaker and Frank, 1948); psychodramatic acting-out (Schindler, 1958); ambivalence towards the therapist (Shellow et al., 1958) negativity, disintegration, distance, disrupted communication—a 'benign regression' (King, 1959) and polarisation with the emergence of sub-groups (Martin and Hill, 1957). On the task level, emotion is expressed as a defence against therapy with challenges to its usefulness and validity (Bach, 1954; Mann and Semrad, 1948; Martin and Hill, 1957). This is a period of extreme resistance to examination and disclosure of information.

Stage three covers the development of cohesion. The emphasis is on consensual group action, co-operation, mutual support (Parker, 1958); integration and mutuality (Mann and Semrad, 1948; Powdermaker and Frank, 1948; Grotjahn, 1950). Members become increasingly aware of the group as a unit; they re-live their family experience or re-experience a new family (Beukenkamp, 1952). This could be called 'pairing' but on a group level, the 'we' stage. Task behaviour is now directed towards discussing oneself and other group members; probing and revealing at an intimate level, confiding, discussing problems in depth (Corsini, 1957; Mann and Semrad, 1948) and exploring individual and group dynamics (Bach, 1954; Martin and Hill, 1957; Powdermaker and Frank, 1948). Transference relationships are particularly apparent in this stage.

The final stage of functional role relatedness on the level of structure is not very evident in psychotherapy groups, but it has been described in terms of the 'use' of cohesion, a period of friendliness and freedom (Corsini, 1957), when emotionality serves rather than impedes a therapeutic function. The group becomes an 'integrative–creative–social instrument' (Martin and Hill, 1957). On the task level, this stage marks the attainment of the group's goal, the emergence of insight into personal and inter-personal processes, and perhaps constructive self-change (cf. Tuckman, 1965).

Summary

Group dynamics is a varied and complex perspective which involves an interdisciplinary approach to the study of group phenomena and draws on extensive academic and professional expertise. Three influential schools of thought within group dynamics have been discussed.

General systems theory, exemplified by Mills's sociological account of group role structure, emphasises the extent to which the behaviour, feelings and ideas expressed by group members are mutually interrelated and shaped by a network of reciprocal expectations which arise from the purposes and functions of the group. Group membership is described as an ongoing participation in gradually more sophisticated roles beginning at the level of interaction and emotion and culminating in a commitment to help determine the norms, goals and values of the group. The theory of family therapy in particular is based on the treatment of the family group as a system with intervention directed at clarifying and modifying the role relationships of family members.

Lewin's *field theory* is founded on a perception of the group as a dynamic whole which occupies a location within an environment and exerts powerful forces inside its own boundaries. This view of the group as a forcefield lends itself to the study of group processes of affiliation and rejection, conformity-inducing pressures and the exercise of power and influence. The field theoretical concept of group cohesiveness is defined as the total of all forces acting upon members to remain in the group, and measures of cohesiveness have been empirically related to outcome in psychotherapy groups. Foulkes's development of group-analytic theory was greatly influenced by Lewin's demonstration of group properties, such as cohesiveness and goals, which could not be reduced to the sum of attributes of individual members.

Finally, Bales's *interaction process analysis* focuses on the investigation of interaction sequences in small groups by means of the elaboration of categories for the classification of both the form and content of interpersonal behaviour. The evidence from process analysis shows that group meetings tend to move through regular patterns of activity which reflect the members' preoccupation with and resolution of the task-related and interpersonal problems posed by the context of interaction. On the task level (what Bion termed the work group), groups are generally characterised by phases of orientation, evaluation and control (i.e. decision-making). These constitute the minimal number of instrumental functions necessary to complete a task. On the social–emotional level (basic assumption group), group activity is successively concentrated on problems of inclusion, authority (dependency) and intimacy (affection). The two levels are dynamically interrelated and the solution of social–emotional problems is a prerequisite for effective work group functioning. Category systems for the analysis of group process have led to more ambitious theories of group development such as Tuckman's comprehensive scheme, in which group members negotiate stages of 'forming, storming, norming and performing'. Awareness of various sequences can alert the group conductor to the important developmental issues facing his group at a specific time in its history.

4 | The mental hospital as a small society

The effect of the overall milieu of the mental hospital on the individual patient has been alluded to in many historical descriptions of the treatment of the mentally ill. Both the physical environment and the psychological environment have been considered. The Egyptians of 2000 BC created temples to which the mentally ill could resort for games and other pastimes. In the first century after Christ, Celsus advised sports, music, reading aloud, rocking in a hammock and the sound of a waterfall, and Caelius Aurelianus about the same era was advising theatricals and entertainments, riding and walking, work discussions and later excursions by land and sea. He also advised, incidentally, that the patient should not see his physician too frequently lest the latter's authority be undermined.

It is probably in the first half of the nineteenth century, however, that the mental hospital environment was more positively and directly invoked as a treatment aid in its own right.

Moral treatment and its aftermath

In the era of moral treatment, as the period from approximately 1800 to 1860 has been described, living conditions in the asylums were being improved. There was undoubtedly an evangelical and religiose fervour about some of the early protagonists of moral treatment, and Samuel Hitch of Gloucester Asylum in 1841 prided himself 'on the extent to which he trusted his patients, putting them on their honour and never refusing a patient's word as a pledge that he would keep a promise' (Rees, 1957). In a similar vein, Browne of the Montrose Royal Lunatic Asylum in 1837 described therein 'a hive of industry', the workers 'loud in their merriment. . . . They literally work in order to please themselves . . . a difficulty is found in restraining their eagerness.' Nevertheless,

'no compulsion, no chains, no whips, no continual chastise-
ment' was necessary in this community because, he goes on, 'these
are proved to be less effectual means of carrying any point than
persuasion, emulation, and the desire of obtaining gratification'.
Charles Dickens, in his *American Notes*, published in 1842, wrote
of the Boston State Hospital:

> Every patient in this asylum sits down to dinner every day
> with a knife and fork and in the midst of them sits the
> gentleman [the Superintendent]. . . . At every meal moral
> influence alone restrains the more violent . . . the effect of
> that influence . . . as a means of restraint, to say nothing of it
> as a means of cure, a hundred times more efficacious than
> all the strait waistcoats, fetters, etc., etc.

At the same time, however, there were a number of remarkably
farsighted physicians who went further than merely to utilise
their personal influence and charisma and who saw the involvement
of patients in the life of the institution as a therapeutic aim rather
than as an economic necessity or a tranquillising diversion. Hack
Tuke, in his *Dictionary of Psychological Medicine* (1892) commences
'If idleness is the curse of the sane, it is the ferment of *ennui* and
mischief to the insane.' He concludes, after reviewing the many
occupations open to the patient in the mental hospital, that 'the
immediate object is not the value of the labour but the benefit of
the patient'. He also notes that 'nursing their fellow patients is a
valuable occupation for both sexes'. The work of Conolly at
Hanwell Asylum was publicised in the *Illustrated London News* of
May 1843, where the employment of patients about the normal
chores of the institution was described, as also were 'large rocking
horses in the airing courts which could accommodate five persons
safely'.

These various activities offered 'a means of amusement and
exercise', says the writer, and 'it may also be said, of an alleviation
of their malady'.

Samuel Woodward, first superintendent of the Worcester State
Hospital (Massachusetts), believed that 'if the physician could
manipulate the environment he could thereby provide the patient
with new and different stimuli; thus older and undesirable patterns
and associations would be broken or modified and new and more
desirable ones substituted in their place' (Grob, 1966). Even earlier
than this, in 1803, Johann Christian Reil of the University of

Halle saw the asylum not as the 'consecrated ground' that Benjamin Rush had regarded it but more realistically as 'the appearance of a stage-show of all of what one has encountered outside' (Harms, 1957). To turn this situation to therapeutic effect he advocated that each asylum should have its own theatre with the roles in the plays 'distributed according to the individual therapeutic needs. The fool, for instance, would be given a role making him aware of the foolishness of his way of behaving, and so on.' Work he saw in graded steps, 'according to the course and progress of the cure', to meet the needs of the patient properly by providing first for physical needs, thence, through artistic activity, to mental activities. And he warned against the 'narrow minded budgetist'. 'Mental institutions, like theatres, are not fit to earn money', he concludes.

The chances of discharge from the mental hospital at this time were quite high, in sharp contrast with what was to follow at the end of the nineteenth century. Thus the discharge rate of patients admitted to the York Retreat within three months of the onset of the illness between the years 1796 and 1861 was about 71 per cent with a very similar figure for the Worcester State Hospital, whereas at the latter institution the overall discharge rate was to fall from 50 per cent in 1830 to 5 per cent in 1880 (Rees, 1957).

On the Continent, particularly in France, Esquirol set the foundations of moral treatment when he stressed the therapeutic function of insane asylums; and Bouchet in 1848 stressed the principle that 'social individuality ought to disappear and merge itself with life in common, which constitutes the real and essential basis for the treatment of the insane' (Rappard et al., 1964). But this psychological orientation was to give way to an increasing reliance on isolation, baths, hypnosis and sedatives.

The latter half of the nineteenth century saw the end of the era of moral treatment. The large institutions deplored by Conolly were now being built to house and contain the accumulating masses of patients that the changing attitudes of society condemned to chronic care. The influence of 'scientific' thinking had led to the belief that mental illness was genetic or due to cellular degeneration and thus incurable. The mentally ill were segregated at some distance from the populace and a feeling of hopelessness pervaded the asylum for both inmates and staff. Discharge was unlikely and escapes a matter of serious concern for the public and the managers, who had to notify such to the Board of Control even until 1924. The whole atmosphere of the asylum became custodial and stagnant.

Summarising the early nineteenth-century experiences, we find many basic truths concerning the social psychology of large residential groups which have since been 're-discovered' by more 'scientific' sociological observation, namely:

(1)   that when the designated leader descends to interact at the level of the common group his power is magnified rather than dissipated;

(2)   that it is not so much the occupation of the group but the active participation in the group activity that is the curative factor;

(3)   that responsibility-sharing and mutual self-help leads to a decrease in passivity and dependence and to abandonment of the sick role; and, conversely,

(4)   that when the aetiology of the illness is placed outside the field of influence of the patient a state of hopelessness is engendered in both therapists and patients;

(5)   that the mental hospital is a microcosm of society with mental symptoms being no more than exaggerations, or acted-out representations, of so-called 'normal' social behaviour;

(6)   that role-playing experiences can lead to insight into the individual's abnormal behaviour; and

(7)   that negative sanctions are less effective than positive reward in changing behaviour.

Something of a return to moral treatment ensued in the decade before World War II when a party of English psychiatrists were much impressed by the freedom from restraints that they witnessed during a tour of mental hospitals in Holland and Germany, particularly at Gutersloh, where Simon had kept alive the nineteenth-century traditions of therapy through involvement in the life of the institution. Work in and around the hospital meant open doors, new communications between staff and patients, with different relationships to be forged, and this called for a reappraisal of the role of the mental nurse (Rees, 1957).

Simon recognised the importance of collaboration between all members of staff for purposes of training and clinical effectiveness. He recommended meetings of doctors, nurses and patients; the holding of common clinical seminars; constant examination of the resistances of both psychiatrist and staff; respect for the patients' defences; and the valuing of patients according to their participation in the hospital. He insisted that the doctor engage himself fully in the study and determination of environmental factors that influenced patient behaviour (Rappard *et al.*, 1964).

The war years finally presented psychiatry with new problems of institutional care in the military psychiatric units where larger groups of young adult neurotics were congregated, and out of these hitherto unprecedented situations new methods of *milieu therapy* arose (see chapter 5). Main (1946), in a paper that described the concept of the hospital as a therapeutic institution, drew on his experience at the Northfield Military Hospital to outline an approach to psychiatric treatment in which the organisation of the hospital and the roles and functions of the staff and patients were radically changed. In this '*therapeutic community*', he described the psychiatrist and the professional staff as members of a community able to contribute opinion from their specialist knowledge towards the resolution of conflict or crisis but no longer directing or managing the life of the patients from a privileged position.

Such an ideal, however, has yet to be attained in its entirety. Traditional roles are for the most part tenaciously held on to by both doctors and patients alike, while bureaucratic administrative policies and general social attitudes restrict the degree to which the old patterns of mental hospital care can be altered. Accounts of the history of the transition from custodial to therapeutic ideology are given by Greenblatt (1960; Greenblatt *et al.*, 1955).

The mental hospital as a social system

Attention was focused on the mental hospital as a social system, i.e. as a particular complex of interacting roles, norms, values and goals, in a series of major studies carried out in the United States (Belknap, 1956; Stanton and Schwartz, 1954; Caudill, 1958; Cumming and Cumming, 1964) and in the UK (Wing and Brown, 1961) in the decade or so following World War II. About the same time, more anecdotal descriptive or philosophic accounts of life in the mental hospital were also published which lent general support to the more scientifically orientated studies (Goffman, 1968; Henry, 1954; Parsons *et al.*, 1953; Barton, 1959). In the main, all of these works emphasised the *deleterious effects* upon the individual of the mental hospital milieu and, in consequence, some efforts were undoubtedly made in psychiatric hospitals to avoid the perpetuation of these adverse conditions. For instance, to avoid institutionalisation there was great pressure to discharge patients as soon as possible to care in the external community, while, to obviate the depersonalising effect of the large institution, psychiatric hospital-building was switched to the production of small acute treatment centres intended to function like general hospital units, to which they were often attached. The associated problems of institutional dependence, depersonalisation, depression and passivity remain with us, however, because they are not primarily problems of the physical environment and thus responsive to structural adjustment but are problems of interpersonal interaction to be understood and remedied by exploration of the group dynamics prevailing in the milieu of the mental patient. In the 1960s and early 1970s a series of papers (e.g. Rockwell, 1971; Stannard, 1973; etc.) continued to report that the main issues of the earlier studies still pertained despite 'the struggle to create a sane society in the psychiatric hospital' (Talbot and Miller, 1966). Indeed, in the seventies an unfortunate series of departmental enquiries into alleged malpractice or negligence in some UK mental hospitals demonstrated that many of the basic situations that had so clearly been shown to lead to stress, conflict, misunderstanding or incidents of violent or disturbed behaviour still maintained relatively unchanged. These were associated with interpersonal behaviour such as poor communication, authoritarian conflicts or staff rivalries rather than inadequate facilities (Report of the Enquiries into St Augustine's Hospital, 1976; Darlington Memorial Hospital, 1976).

Some of the main problems for the mental hospital community arise out of the unresolved issue as to what the primary function of the mental hospital should be (Moos, 1974). Conflict of aims is generated between the objective of 'curing' the patient for his benefit or 'controlling' the patient for the benefit of the society that has committed him to the hospital. Bott (1976) showed how the hospital's divided responsibility to individual patients and to society (relatives and others) led to intrinsic strain within the hospital, particularly among staff and even within individual staff members. Parsons (1951b) has described the social organisation that arises in the mental hospital as being that of a governor and the governed rather than a server and the served. Goffman (1968) has gone a step further and analysed the server–served metaphor, which he found quite inapplicable to the actual expertise psychiatry can offer and the source of many difficulties with which psychiatric hospitals must contend.

The prevailing attitude in the mental hospital milieu to which the individual patient becomes subjected on admission is inevitably dependent upon and influenced by the attitude of and prevailing public opinion in the wider society outside the mental hospital which fluctuates periodically between understanding and a liberal outlook and uncertainty and restriction so that, in one decade, patients are urged to mix freely with the outside community while in the next the hospital authorities are called upon to provide more constraints and, indeed, security units. Bott (1976) has suggested that these uncertainties and fluctuations are basically about the social location of madness and depend on the extent to which society, in any historical period, is prepared to accept a more permeable boundary between the 'insane' and the 'sane'.

The studies and their findings

Stanton and Schwartz (1954) made an intensive survey of Chestnut Lodge Sanitorium in the United States which was a privately run mental hospital with a psychotherapeutic orientation. With these provisos in mind, however, the majority of their findings can be applied to other mental hospitals. Caudill (1958) similarly studied hospital organisation through the device of being admitted as a patient and collaborating with a staff sociologist, and Cumming and Cumming (1964) both explored the system and attempted to incorporate the socio-dynamics into a coherent milieu therapy approach. They saw the *ego* as developing through resolution of a series of graded situations of conflict provided by the milieu, much as Erikson (1950) has described the normal development of personality through the facing and overcoming of crises of increasing complexity with the passage of the years. Goffman's (1968) more anecdotal and highly critical account of 'asylums' was gathered from observations made from a pseudo-staff role as a gymnasium assistant which he then generalised to other 'total institutions' where a subject group is stripped of personality and individuality by the controlling group.*

The Wing and Brown (1961) study was of three English mental hospitals where the social conditions and attitudes prevailing were

---

*Kesey (1962), who had worked briefly as a night attendant at an Oregon Mental Hospital, transferred his not dissimilar impressions into the novel and film, *One Flew Over the Cuckoo's Nest*.

investigated with reference to the behaviour of the longer-term schizophrenic patients. At the hospital where there was interest in, and emphasis on, the long-stay patient, there was least clinical disturbance and most personal freedom (e.g. to retain possessions) with useful occupations and optimism among the nursing staff. At another hospital, where throughout the institution there were still features of 'the bad old mental hospital', such as padded rooms, side rooms used for seclusion, with ECT and sedation used to control disturbed behaviour instead of active occupation, there was most clinical disturbance among patients, least personal freedom and useful occupation and least optimism among staff. The third hospital came somewhat in between in both the findings and the steps that had been taken toward a more progressive outlook. The conclusions were cautious but suggested that social conditions can and do influence the state of schizophrenic patients.

The effects of the mental hospital milieu

The *collective findings* of the studies referred to above and the related papers can be summarised as follows.

(a) On symptom formation and patient behaviour

The environment itself may be the cause of the symptoms. Thus, Stanton and Schwartz (1954) described manic excitement resulting from staff disagreements on the ward so that the emotional atmosphere in which the patient finds himself is highly charged, uncertain and volatile, and he, the most vulnerable group member, responds accordingly. Henry (1954) similarly points out that when ward staff are exposed to different treatment ideologies by their various superiors tension and confusion is generated within them and passed down to the patient level. Behaviour that is unacceptable and inappropriate in a normal setting may have real meaning and be all that is left for the patient to express himself by in the emotionally and materially deprived situation of the mental hospital. Thus, Stanton and Schwartz (1954) refer to incontinence as a final aggression in the patient confined to bed and Goffman (1968) to faecal smearing in the padded cell where all other communication materials are denied the patient. Disturbed behaviour in the mental hospital gains the attention of the staff and thus, paradoxically, is rewarded, while the quiescent patient can be overlooked and ignored. Passive acceptance of the norms of the institution, however, finally comes to be looked upon as good behaviour likely to lead to discharge (Main, 1946). The patient may have to surrender somewhat to the staff structure in order to gain his discharge (Goffman, 1968) but he must not proclaim his improvement too earnestly lest he is dismissed as unrealistic! (Caudill, 1958). In his treatise on *Institutional Neurosis*, Barton (1959) described the induced apathy and passivity in the long-term mental hospital patient, under-stimulated and socially neglected, which itself became the greatest handicap to reabsorption into the outside community when the symptoms of the illness for which the patient was originally hospitalised had long since remitted.

(b) On staff attitudes and behaviour

Good leadership is essential. The chain of influence is described by Belknap (1956) passing down the hierarchichal line from medical superintendent to ward orderly and into the patient level. It is usually the junior ward staff who spend most time with the patients, and yet these will be the least well trained and generally the poorest emotionally equipped for the task by reason of their youth and lack of experience or knowledge. Their role is a difficult one. Lacking status, they have few institutionalised defences to hide behind. They do not carry the same protection as does the respected doctor or ward sister in the treater-and-treated interaction.

If communications and contacts between the ward staff and the patients have been opened up by a 'progressive' therapeutic programme then it is the anxieties of the lowly ward staff that will be most raised. Feeling threatened, they may retreat into defensive positions out of contact with the patients, such as busying themselves with the linen room or in the ward office. Cohler and Shapiro (1964) call such defences 'avoidance patterns' and distinguish withdrawal, acting-out through patients and over-involvement arising from identification with the patients. Leckwart (1968) put forward the view that the social distance between staff members and patients, that is the degree of closeness or intimacy that characterises their day-to-day interactions, has a decisive influence on the effectiveness of a 'helping relationship'. Defensive withdrawal leads to extreme social distancing, which can seriously jeopardise the realisation of treatment aims. Similar comments on this theme are made by Bockoven (1963); Henry (1954); Schwartz and Shockley (1956); and Schwartz and Will (1953). When an atmosphere of permissiveness has been implemented from above the patients will push and test out the limits increasing the stresses on the ward staff. One result may be that, at ward level, staff feeling anxious and threatened may enter into a self-protective and collusive alliance with the patients against the nominal policy from above (Goffman, 1968). Main (1957) initiated group discussions among nursing staff to deal with the emotional roots of collusive relationships. Burnham (1966) has reviewed the literature on this important problem, and he delineated a complex relationship between staff members and 'special problem' patients, who were simultaneously victims and agents of splitting processes. Thus, the more 'progressive', 'liberal' or 'democratic' the regime, the more essential it becomes for the stable, secure and ideologically committed senior staff to be seen on or about the ward, and involved in the newly created emotional life of the ward group. The importance of involvement for senior staff themselves has been highlighted by several studies that examined the effects on staff of their position in the status hierarchy. Mishler and Trapp (1956) found that, the greater the status differential between staff members, the less they interacted. This finding can be extended to include interactions with patients. Both Sheldrake and Turner (1963) and Whiting and Murray (1961) suggested that staff members' perceptions were influenced by status; for example, in the former study the higher a nurse was in the status hierarchy, the more her perception of a patient–nurse relationship differed from the patient's perception.

On the other hand, staff who interpret their role as merely to observe and report to superiors who will be responsible for the treatment may come to regard the most normal acts as pathological in a patient who has been labelled as mentally abnormal. Thus, requesting a glass of water may be logged as a 'therapeutic' communication worthy of comment (Stanton and Schwartz, 1954). Rockwell (1971), who as a junior psychiatrist exposed himself to a brief sojourn in the role of a patient, reported on the paranoia-inducing effect of such impersonal scrutiny. The reality world of the patient can be overlooked by the staff engaged in seeking out the pathology or meaning behind the patient's thought, words and deeds.

Even when staff behaviour towards patients is not manifestly the result of defensive reactions, staff are bound to interact differentially with patients according to their liking or preference for particular kinds of patients. Morgan and Cheadle (1972), for example, found that if a group of patients is rank-ordered in terms of preference or rejection by staff, a sub-group of relatively rejected patients was bound to appear. A similar unpublished study carried out at the Henderson Hospital showed that patients who were considered threatening or who aroused anger in staff also made staff feel they were 'getting nowhere' with these patients. This implies that if, on admission, a patient is consigned to the lower positions of an implicit preference rank order, his treatment career may be crucially affected. One of the functions of clinical leadership is systematically to make these value judgements and subjective responses explicit.

A variety of differing treatment approaches and ideologies in the one institution can lead to confusion and deterioration in function, as Kotin and Sharas (1967) described; and adherence to one ideological approach, whatever it is—physical or psychological—is more productive than diverse and often conflicting approaches and ideologies. Thus, once again, clear and decisive leadership from above is called for with resolution of ideological conflicts at the highest level as an essential to good functioning throughout the institution.

Just as staff need to know where they stand, what is expected of them and what they may expect of each other person in the group that constitutes the mental hospital milieu, so do the patients. For both, the locked security ward can, paradoxically, sometimes be the least stressful, for here limits have been set up. Staff and patients know their positions and within the defined limits there may be greater personal freedom then in other situations where expectations and rules are less rigidly spelled out (Stanton and Schwartz, 1954).

(c) On the two-tier structure of the mental hospital

While conceptualising the mental hospital as one encapsulated large group, it is nevertheless important to recognise within that group the two distinct sub-groups of the patients and the staff with little movement or transaction across that interface except in a strictly 'therapeutic' interaction. When staff become ill they are usually admitted to another hospital for treatment, and when recovered patients seek psychiatric work they will usually be referred to another institution to seek employment.

Loeb (1956) described the two-tier culture of the mental hospital as being 'the haves' and the 'have nots', symbolically referring to the key of the ward but also to the freedom, privileges, status and, indeed, rights to lead a normal life possessed by the one group and denied to the other. Goffman (1968), in particular, describes vividly how the patient group then develops its own protective under-life in the institution, denying access to the staff group, who in turn have denied access to their group to the patient group. Rowland (1938) describes the defensive alliance of the patients in order to withstand the hospital structure, and Talbot *et al.* (1964) describes the way that hospitalised patients quickly retreat into regressive, 'sick', socially disturbed behaviour in the hospital transacting with the staff through a series of socially abnormal or inappropriate acts which have come to be regarded as meaningful by staff working in a psychotherapeutic orientation. The reality world of the individual in his immediate environment is lost sight of by both sides.

The life and death of a mental hospital

A study by Stotland and Kobler (1965) under the above title graphically described the cumulative effects of the social forces and group processes at work in the milieu of a mental hospital such as have been outlined in this chapter, and this is worth summarising.

The small, privately funded hospital was set up with high hopes and founded on a form of milieu therapy in the 1950s. Early rivalry between the staff leaders and ideological differences among them and between them and the Committee of Management was reflected down the chain of command to ward level. Tensions arose, particularly about the use of physical treatments or psychotherapy. Staff morale decreased and one of the staff leaders broke down and had to leave. Succeeding leaders were invested with impossibly high expectations or faced with outright antagonism until they too became entrenched in positions of isolated authority or broke down into deviant or neglectful behaviour. The discord spread through the staff. Personal and professional behaviour deteriorated, and the nursing aides held a wild and scandalous party. Then the adolescent patients acted-out in a rebellion against

95

treatment, pushing at the uncertain limits. This was dealt with by an excess of authoritarian discharges. ECT became more extensively used, as if to reassert the influence and control that the nurses no longer felt they held on the wards, and then a rash of suicides followed as the patients, too, lost hope in the treatment process. Finally the hospital had to close.

Constructing the treatment environment

Goffman (1968) has commented on the inappropriateness of the mental hospital modelled on the medical approach for the treatment of mental illness. He says that a mental hospital is ill-equipped to be a place where a classic *repair* cycle occurs (i.e. a place where a defect or breakdown is corrected), for the staff are largely engaged in the observation or recording of deviant behaviour rather than in performing a reparative function.

Main (1946) doubted whether the mental hospital could remain a building within which individual treatment along psycho-therapeutic lines could be usefully undertaken. He advocated that treatment of the emotionally disturbed individual, who suffered from a disturbance of social relationships, should be undertaken within a framework of *social reality*, where real responsibilities were put before the patient and the staff were servants of the community rather than controlling agents. Only in this way could the hospital become a therapeutic institution.

Psychotherapy in the mental hospital setting has been described by Talbot *et al.* (1964) as anti-therapeutic in the way that it can encourage a group regression to abnormal, acting-out types of 'sick' communication; and Maxwell Jones (1956), in an early paper on the therapeutic community, emphasised that the aim of the 'therapeutic community' in the mental hospital would be the adjustment of the individual to social and work conditions outside, 'without any ambitious psychotherapeutic programme'. The inference is that psychotherapy can encourage a resort to fantasy life and unconscious preoccupations and thus has little place in the reality of the living situation in the mental hospital.

Edelson (1970) separates psychotherapy and sociotherapy, keeping the processes quite distinct in his treatment approach. *Psychotherapy* is seen as directed at the internal state of the patient, and it is Edelson's opinion that psychotherapeutic interventions in the large group meeting are obstructive and anti-therapeutic. He confines such to separate psychotherapeutic sessions conducted with the patient individually or in small analytic groups. *Sociotherapy* is described as directed at the social setting in which the patient is resident, and the sociotherapist is restricted to observing, clarifying and facilitating where appropriate the major social processes that Edelson identifies in the large hospital or ward group. These are the processes that deal with problems of:

(1) integration (e.g. of new members);
(2) adaptation (e.g. to new situations);
(3) consummation (i.e. of desired objectives); and
(4) motivation (i.e., the expression of aims and purposes).

Such a distinction between sociotherapy and psychotherapy as applied to the mental hospital milieu or the ward group is not held by everyone, however. Tosquelles (1964) of the French Institutional Therapy movement conceives of the hospital as a blend of sociological and psychological concepts. 'If, in psychoanalysis,' he says,

it is the doctor who is the object of successive investments and transference fantasies, in the therapeutic institution it is the social life itself which is the object of these investments. It is not sufficient therefore, to multiply activities and to develop a material mastery of the milieu; social structures of themselves have no curative power but they are the framework for multiple unconscious processes of dramatic identification and it is within these social networks that the doctor must work.

Recent trends in the mental health situation point more urgently to the need to develop adequate skills for working in the milieu of the mental hospital. Although overall population figures in the hospital are decreasing slightly and the numbers of new admissions for the major psychoses are declining, there is a marked increase in the admissions for alcoholism and personality disorder, both of which are conditions more clearly rooted in disturbance of the social environment and interpersonal behaviour of the patient (Statistical and Research Report, 1973). Moreover, the new long-stay patients—the ones who stay from one to five years—are people who, in addition to their basic illness (schizophrenia in two-thirds of the cases), have marked social handicaps such as social isolation or occupational inadequacy (Mann, 1975). For most of these, the hospital and particularly the newer form of general hospital psychiatric unit geared to acute treatment, quick turnover and physical therapies, is quite inadequate. Indeed, it could be argued that 'hospital' treatment of any kind is inappropriate and a more socially orientated management in a hostel or community home would more adequately meet their needs.

The issues for the mental hospital community are thus:

(1) *To define the aim of the milieu.* If *control* and *cure* are two sometimes conflicting functions a third—*care*—of the long-stay patient with social handicaps is becoming of increasing importance. It is necessary for the hospital to provide for all of these three needs appropriately and without confusion of purpose.

(2) *To implement the aims.* In the WHO Technical Report of the Expert Committee on Mental Health (1953) it is reported that

> the most important single factor in the efficacy of treatment given in a mental hospital appears to the Committee to be an intangible element which can only be described as its atmosphere . . . as in the community at large one of the characteristic aspects of the psychiatric hospital is the type of relationship between the people that are to be found within it; the nature of the relationship between the medical director and his staff will be reflected in the relationship between the psychiatric staff and the nurses and finally in the relationship not only between the nurses and the patients but between the patients themselves.

Decisive leadership, clear ideological aims, open communication of the theoretical aspects of the treatment and the capacity to resolve issues of conflict within the staff group are important for the efficient functioning of the hospital as a controlling, caring or curing milieu. Staff training and the involvement of staff of all disciplines in the therapeutic function of the milieu will sharpen the treatment focus.

The splintering of the staff personnel into groupings with wholly unintegrated functions, or even rival purposes, destroys the possibility of a functioning milieu process. Ideally, the administrators, the maintenance men, cooks and cleaners, as well as the traditional treatment staff should be seen as part of the milieu with a therapeutic function to perform. The shedding of the treatment responsibility on to the professional staff alone, and in actual practice largely on to the doctors, leaves untapped a vast resource of human potential in the role of ancillary staff, ward aides, junior nurses and other para-medical staff who interpret their job as, mainly, to observe and report, and who defer to the doctor in the area of treatment. The influx of overseas doctors and nurses with real barriers of language and culture must have an effect on the process of communication and empathy.

Awareness of the well documented, adverse effects of the mental hospital milieu, is of first importance, intruding as they do into all the three stated aims of the mental hospital. The generation of positive therapeutic processes through the utilisation of the inherent milieu forces follows. The curative aspects of therapy through the milieu are dealt with more fully in chapter 5, but in the general mental hospital, dealing with heterogeneous problems and cases and with its acknowledged diverse aims and limitations, the milieu can be still made to work as a therapeutic tool.

The mental hospital environment

The three main areas of the mental hospital patient's life are in the *ward*, the *workshop* and the *recreational* areas. These distinct areas, often geographically separate entities with different staff composition and carrying different expectations and role performance, are embraced within the totality of the hospital. Thrasher and Smith (1964) also distinguished several types of interactional context (ward, patient society and cliques) which each tended to generate different patient behaviours. The whole affects the parts and the parts affect the whole.

The *physical environment* that the hospital provides is of secondary importance to the emotional environment engendered by the staff and the staff leaders. Nevertheless, its constraints, inadequacies and architectual design will direct treatment in one or another way and even make impossible some treatment approaches. Thus, the hospital designed as an acute treatment unit will make it virtually impossible to contain the excited psychotic, the elderly dement or the acting-out adolescent. Such problem cases need space to move around in, self-contained living areas for easy orientation, or physical activity opportunities, for example. The psychiatric ward attached to the general hospital usually determines that the course of treatment follows the medical model of the parent hospital with pharmacological therapy, sedation, bedrest and restraints upon physical and emotional expression.

The design and furnishing of a psychiatric unit likewise exerts an effect on the milieu in which the patient is treated. Revulsion for the degrading surroundings of many backward mental hospitals has led to their replacement with hotel-like comforts in some hospital-building programmes, yet the new environments have brought no particular improvement in behaviour (Polansky *et al.*, 1957; Cumming and Cumming, 1964). The surroundings provided have been inappropriate to the post-discharge expectations and reality environments of the patients and as such can be strange and unaccustomed appurtenances leading in their turn to feelings of inappropriateness and unreality. Furnishings and fittings need to be of an ordinary type to which the patient is accustomed in his daily life and with which he is at ease. The mystique and specialness of hospital buildings should be minimised but where doors are locked and access restricted, a notice should explain the reason why. A patient in our hospital spent his first two anxious days going round every room in the vast dilapidated building opening doors and cupboards and going through every room like an animal apprehensively exploring a cage. Helping the patient to physically locate himself in the environment helps him toward the reassumption of his real identity and self-image. Thus, ward reception and an introduction to fellow patients and to ward staff with a tour of the building has a socio-therapeutic purpose. Disturbed behaviour, often violence to staff, can easily result when a patient is moved from one ward to another without adequate communication as to the reason why or careful preparation.

The ward

Frequent staff changes on the ward destroy the possibility of familiar and easy relationships building up between staff and patients, while the dispersal of the patients to different parts of the hospital for 'treatment', 'testing', 'social work interview' or 'recreation' prevent the building up of an involvement with the ward and its milieu and thus the development of identifications.

Small and self-contained units within the hospital, with social, recreational, occupational and general living activities under the one roof, as it were, are paradoxically found only on the disturbed ward, and not for the therapeutic potential, which is enormous, but for reasons of security and segregation from the 'normal' parts of the hospital, which, because of their very diverse and specialist functions, are the most unlike a normal living situation.

In the pursuit of a physical environment not like a hospital and 'just like outside', however, one must be aware of the anxieties that can be provoked in already confused patients in unusual surroundings if they are surrounded by masses of strange people and expected to eat, socialise and sleep in large 'integrated' groups of both sexes, and if they cannot locate the nursing attendants because, in a misguided belief that uniforms are necessarily bad and that normal clothes should be worn by the staff, the nurse is indistinguishable from all other people on the ward.

In a gesture towards the revelations of Stanton and Schwartz, the Cummings, Caudill and others, and attempting to emulate the therapeutic community practice of Main and Maxwell Jones, most psychiatric hospitals instituted ward meetings in the early days of socio-therapeutic awareness. The tradition continues, but in many cases has become institutionalised and lost its function. The practitioners are unaware of the real dynamics of the group and unskilled in their management, and patients are confused as to the aims and purpose. The ward meeting is often no more than a grumble session about the cold morning tea or the lateness of the medication trolley. The ward sister presides, with arms akimbo as the junior doctor on duty grapples embarrassingly with the complaints. If a psychotic patient interrupts the proceedings the nurses immediately remove him or, as one doctor explained, 'we ignore him'. Since the psychotic communication is more than likely a protest against the non-acknowledgement by his fellows, abnormal behaviour can only be exaggerated until he gets a response.

Hall (1973) reviews the literature on the ward as an entity in itself.

The *ward meeting* should be seen in the overall context of the social organisation within which it is located (Jones, 1966), i.e., the mental hospital, and not as an isolated large group for primarily psychoanalytic interventions and interpretations. A study of ward behaviour relative to the existence of ward meetings in the psychiatric unit of a general hospital (Maratos and Kennedy, 1974) showed that behaviour improved in terms of there being less communication through acting-out when ward meetings were held and that this was a direct effect of having the opportunity for free expression and unrelated to psychotherapeutic direction or intervention or even to a positive attitude from the ward staff towards the meeting. Perhaps the most important aspect of the ward meeting is the sharing of problems with patients, comment Jones and Hollingsworth (1963a), and helping them find ways of dealing more effectively with their everyday crises. Continuity of membership is important; and attendance and participation by all members of the staff team is necessary for full exploration of the interpersonal problems, real and fantasised, as they arise; and frequency of meetings is essential if actual day-to-day problems are to be explored. Ideally, the daily ward meeting of all staff and patients lasting sixty minutes, unstructured except perhaps for a neutral chairman who acts as 'gate-keeper', opening and closing the meeting, excluding material that should properly be dealt with elsewhere (e.g. how another ward should be run) will allow the gradual development of conflict situations into the form in which they can be explored or resolved (Jones and Hollingsworth, 1963b). The fluctuations in mood, the cycles of organisation and disorganisation (Rapoport, 1960), the moves towards independence or towards regression and dependency will then take their normal turn over the days and weeks, and the more permanent members of the group (i.e., the staff) will be in a position to point out the prevailing social dynamics, the effect on the group members and the ways in which resolution can be achieved.

The workshop

Occupational therapy in the mental hospital has a long tradition but its rise as specialist function to some extent destroyed the working parties that had traditionally gone about the business of restoring or refurbishing the physical milieu of the hospital. Such working parties would often be in the charge of artisans rather than therapists, but the human relationships that developed therein, as each respected the other for his skill or adequacy at the task, were valued treatment aspects. The rise of separateness and job specification in the mental hospital resulted in the loss of this facet of the treatment. Cumming and Cumming (1964) suggest that it is always best if there is something left to do in the physical environment of the hospital, in which the patients can be occupied, either physically, to achieve the desired result, or intellectually and executively, in deciding what is to be done.

Maxwell Jones commented that it was perhaps fortunate that the original Belmont (later Henderson Hospital) was in such a poor condition because it gave the patients scope for involvement in the task of upgrading their surroundings. Pride in the results follows and there is less destruction of what would otherwise be anonymous hospital property.

Industrial therapy had its vogue in the mid-1960s in an attempt to introduce long-stay patients to the realities of factory life, thus fitting them for life outside the hospital. The concentration on work schedules and a relative refusal to look at the interpersonal aspects of the working group has been an unsuccessful venture. Poor output, in quantity and quality, has resulted in fewer contracts being gained and the work itself becoming of the most menial and soul-destroying type. Concentration on the interpersonal aspects of the workshop lessens the industrial output still further but, as Miles (1972) described in a controlled comparison of an orthodox workshop under the direction of industrial staff and one run on therapeutic community lines, where the patients themselves were cast in the roles of foreman, instructors, progress-chaser etc., the social awareness and interpersonal connections and communications increased significantly in the therapeutic community-orientated group. The true function of the mental hospital workshop is surely to produce personality improvement, not saleable goods.

Social therapy

The aspect in which mental hospital patients are most inadequate will often be that of socialising with other people (McCowen and Wilder, 1975), and this is even less than the workshop regarded as a treatment area. Yet, as Rowland pointed out as early as 1938: 'The fact of the matter is that the mental patient must associate every day with other mental patients. From the sociological standpoint, this is of greater importance than all other aspects of life in the mental hospital.'

The provision of entertainments in an institutional way serves only to occupy or divert the patient but gives him no opportunity for developing social skills.

Involvement of the patients in formalised roles within the hospital—as members of the entertainments committee, patients' reception group, visitors' orientation programme, etc.—allows social roles to be played out and unaccustomed behaviour to be attempted, provided it is also understood that commentary upon the role-functioning will be a part of the contract. This means staff participation in the social and living situation of the hospital and the provision of 'after-group' sessions in which free comment on each other's performance is permissible. Actual role-playing of social engagements or employment situations can be introduced, and when social events are held within the hospital or ward both preparatory and post-mortem discussions can explore the desired and actual behaviour of the participants. Hall (1973) comments:

> socialisation continues to take place as long as the patient is continuing to make progress toward discharge. He is constantly being socialised into more and more complicated roles on the ward and he is constantly refining and testing in the social sphere his beliefs about ways of adjusting to life on the ward and in the world.

Conclusions

In the period following World War II the milieu and the function of the mental hospital in the mental health services has changed significantly—not in any dramatic way but rather insidiously.

The staff have splintered into sub-groups with little unification of purpose, roles have defined rather than blurred into the common therapeutic task, and the interest and impetus of treatment has been taken into extramural activities and projects. The influx of overseas staff at all levels has inevitably brought real difficulties of communication and cultural misunderstanding. All of these factors have considerably decreased the positive aspects of the hospital milieu while increasing the possibility for the emergence of the ill effects of the milieu.

On the patient side the changes have been towards the accumulation of people with problems of social maladaption and for whom the milieu is of particular importance.

It becomes of increasing rather than decreasing importance, therefore, for the staff working in mental hospitals to be aware of the negative effects and the positive potential of the milieu in psychiatric treatment.

The concept of the therapeutic community

The term 'therapeutic community' is one of the most misused and misunderstood terms in modern psychiatry. It has been used to describe the treatment attitude of whole hospitals and the specific regime of certain wards for problematical patients. After-care hostels, penal establishments and day centres have all been so described, and it is this widespread use of the term that has given credence to critics such as Zeitlyn (1967), who pointed out the gaps between ideology and practice, or Harrington (1970), who, after pointing out some of the contradictions and paradoxes in a therapeutic community, doubted if it had any scientific validity and was really anything more than a humanitarian approach to mental treatment.

Abroms (1969) has used the term 'metatherapy' to describe a context within which various treatment modalities and techniques, including pharmacological, behavioural, individual psychotherapy and group processes of all kinds, are systematically organised and utilised to meet specific treatment goals. This technology goes beyond the humanistic values of moral treatment. We take the view that the therapeutic community is a specific, specialised treatment process, utilising the psychological and sociological phenomena inherent in the large, circumscribed and residential group. In this respect it is an intensified extension of milieu therapy as described in the preceeding chapter, which has more general implications and applications for patients of all categories in the mental hospital community.

In order to understand the therapeutic community in this specific way it is necessary to study the course of its development in psychiatry.

Origins

In so far as psychiatry is concerned, the origins were in the military neurosis units of World War II in the United Kingdom followed by similar experiences in the United States (Wilmer, 1958) when the war brought to them identical problems. In the decade prior to the war psychiatrists such as Harry Stack Sullivan (1931) and the Menningers (1939) had drawn attention to the social dynamics of the hospital ward and group therapy itself was coming into being. There was an inclination in psychiatry, and indeed among the newer psychoanalysts such as Fromm and Horney, to take more notice of social and cultural factors in the aetiology of neurosis.

Outside of psychiatry, educationists and youth workers had, since the early part of the century, employed 'living and learning' situations to replace deviant and maladjusted behaviour with more socially acceptable conduct. Makarenko and the Gorki Republics in Russia, Father Flanagan and Boys' Town in the United States and Homer Lane and the Little Commonwealth in England are historic examples of self-governing communities where roles were played out, behaviour examined by the group and new methods of inte-grated and co-operative functioning explored (Whiteley et al., 1972). Initially, these experiments were very much in the model of social control by group processes, but as the 1920s and 1930s proceeded a more psychological and frankly psychoanalytical influence was incorporated which, in inexperienced hands, led to disaster as with Homer Lane, for example. Marjorie Franklin, a psychoanalyst, and David Wills, a teacher, were more successful in the enterprise with Q camps which were residential camps for delinquent boys, and out of this experience was formulated a project of Planned Environment Therapy (Righton, 1975).

Psychiatry, however, generally remained aloof from these progressive strivings until the new situation created by wartime neurosis casualties called for an innovative treatment approach. In contrast to the heterogeneity of the civilian mental hospital popula-tion, the military neurosis units brought together young adults of similar age span and similar neurotic disorder, which was a dis-order rooted in a similar *social* aetiology, namely the disruption of their lives by the military experience, and out of this situation *two* treatment approaches emerged.

The Northfield experiment

In the attempt to meet the new problems of the management of emotionally disturbed combatants more constructively than had been the case in World War I, when large numbers of such patients had been categorised as 'shell-shocked', became useless to the war effort and were trapped thenceforward by pension allocation and public regard into longstanding disability in the mistaken belief that they were organically injured, the Tavistock Clinic was called upon for advice. In a short-lived experiment of six to eight weeks W. R. Bion, a psychologist and psychoanalyst of Kleinian orientation, took the far-sighted step of viewing his ward as a group rather than as individuals and seeing the neurotic behaviour of the ward inmates as an unconscious alliance between them in this special situation in relation to the hospital, the military authority and the problems surrounding them. His acceptance of the situation, and his permitting its continuation through stages of regression until some resolution might emerge from the group, was not appreciated by the powers that be and the experiment was terminated. He later drew on the observations and conceptualisations of this important period in the opening chapters of his classic work, *Experiences in Groups* (Bion, 1961). He was followed by a succession of psychiatrists, most of whom had psychoanalytic training or interest and who developed on Bion's innovative approach, seeing the hospital as a functioning whole made up of dynamically interacting units. Problems affecting the whole would be reflected by various disturbances in the parts, and problems arising in a part would affect the well-being of the whole. Foulkes and Anthony (1957) described this as the Second Northfield Experiment to distinguish it from Bion's approach, and this time the concept flourished. Out of this experience Main (1946) coined the term 'therapeutic community' and described in an article in the *Bulletin* of the Menninger Clinic in 1946 the prerequisites of 'the hospital as a therapeutic institution'. He wrote:

> The Northfield Experiment is an attempt to use a hospital
> not as an organisation run by doctors in the interests of their
> own greater technical efficiency, but as a community with the
> immediate aim of full participation of all its members in its
> daily life and the eventual aim of the resocialisation of the
> neurotic individual for life in ordinary society. Ideally, it has
> been conceived as a therapeutic setting with a spontaneous
> and emotionally structured (rather than medically dictated)
> organisation in which all staff and patients engage. Any
> attempt to permit or create such a setting demands tolerance,

a willingness to profit by error, and a refusal to jump to conclusions; but certain matters appear to be plain. The daily life of the community must be related to real tasks, truly relevant to the needs and aspirations of the small society of the hospital, and the larger society in which it is set; there must be no barriers between the hospital and the rest of society; full opportunity must be available for identifying and analysing the interpersonal barriers which stand in the way of participation in a full community life.

These are not small requirements and they have demanded a review of our attitudes as psychiatrists towards our own status and responsibilities. The anarchical rights of the doctor in the traditional hospital society have to be exchanged for the more sincere role of member in a real community, responsible not only to himself and his superiors, but to the community as a whole, privileged and restricted only insofar as the community allows or demands. He no longer owns 'his' patients. They are given up to the community which is to treat them, and which owns them and him. Patients are no longer his captive children, obedient in nursery-like activities, but have sincere adult roles to play, and are free to reach for responsibilities and opinions concerning the community of which they are a part. They, as well as he, must be free to discuss a rationale of daily hospital life, to identify and analyse the problems, formulate the conditions and forge the enthusiasms of group life. The patients must be free to plan and organise activities of actual hospital procedure, and thus face together problems of immediate social reality. Failures of organisation, internal problems of apathy, insecurity, and hostility, as well as ordinary practical difficulties are matters for solution by the patients who own the community and create the problems.

Foulkes (Foulkes and Anthony, 1957) described his own work at Northfield as 'essentially analytical', which gives some clue as to how the work was carried out. The role of the therapist at Northfield was to sit in on the activities of the hospital wards and workshops, to observe and to interpret behaviour and to facilitate the resolution of problems as they became apparent or as the group sought help. Sometimes the advice would be quite directive, as Foulkes describes in the exclusion of a trouble-making patient from a particular group. Foulkes also says that Northfield might well be called the nursery of British group analysis and that 'because of the Northfield experience and its great impetus group analysis in Britain took a wholly independent line from America and in the group sense was more advanced'.

Main (1946) describes for the therapist a varied but skilled and specialist role 'as a technician among, rather than a superintendent of his patients'. The aim of the Northfield unit (and subsequent therapeutic communities) was

> a socialisation of neurotic drives, their modification by social demands within a real setting, the ego-strengthening, the increased capacity for sincere and easy social relationships, and the socialisation of super-ego demands to provide the individual with a capacity and a technique for stable life in a real role in the real world'.

Out of this particular conceptualisation of a therapeutic community with its undoubted leaning toward psychoanalytic theory and practice, despite its social intent, there emerged a type of therapeutic community with psychoanalytic orientation which was carried over after the war into the treatment of neurotics at units like the Cassel Hospital and Ingrebourne Centre. Crocket (1960, 1962) and others (Tollinton, 1969) at the latter unit have more specifically defined the process as a *psycho-therapeutic community*, wherein boundaries are set for patient or staff activity, roles are fairly well determined and limits are set between what behaviour is permissible and what is not. The staff, and particularly the staff leader, retain the responsibility for the overall process of treatment, the timing of specific events, such as progress from the introductory group to a further group or to discharge, and the type of events that will occur in the treatment course.

The Mill Hill development

Simultaneously with the developments at Northfield, a similar situation presented itself at the Military Neurosis Unit at Mill Hill where Maxwell Jones, with a background of more 'medically' orientated psychiatry from the Maudsley Hospital, headed a treatment team. The early papers by Maxwell Jones stress the need to communicate information in an authoritative way, and he embarked upon a system of lecturing to the patients as if to medical students, explaining the origin of psychosomatic symptoms by reference to physiological and anatomical diagrams. This didactic method soon gave way to a dialogue when members of the audience asked questions or volunteered other than medical theories as to the origin of their problems. The dialogue between patient and doctor gave way in its turn to open discussion by the 'class' and the problems of everyday living in the hospital became pertinent topics for discussion and resolution in the large group forum that developed. Thus, while Northfield was a consciously set up *experiment*, the Mill Hill community *evolved* according to the expressed needs of those concerned. Although the two projects and what was to develop from them overlap considerably, they were different in origin, in practice and indeed in aim. Maxwell Jones subsequently utilised the same principles developed at Mill Hill namely large group discussion, open communication, flattening of the hierarchical pyramid and role-blurring, to facilitate the resolution of problems arising in other communities by the group members themselves. He turned his attention particularly to those problems that more clearly had roots in a disturbance of the social system of the individual. Thus he tackled the problems of the returning prisoner-of-war— 'displaced'—in many real or fantasised ways in society, employment, marriage and family. Later he turned to the problems of the seemingly industrially misplaced, employing with them, as with the POW's, a 'total push' approach, which exposed them to a variety of social situations, training courses and interpersonal skills. Gradually this superficially 'social' approach gave way to the introduction of psychological or psychoanalytic techniques or theories (he himself embarked upon a personal psychoanalysis about this time) as he and his colleagues came to accept that 'displacement' in society was not necessarily due wholly to lack of opportunity or experience but also owed much to deficits of personality functioning. The emotionally unsettled individual would be emotionally unsettled in response to any situation, and environmental change alone would have little effect on his behaviour.

When the unit at Belmont (Rapoport, 1960) was renamed the Social Rehabilitation Unit in 1952 the emphasis was now on inadequacy of role-functioning in the family and in society, and the exploratory and treatment techniques were more clearly aligned to the social psychiatry studies that Stanton and Schwartz (1954) and Caudill (1958) were now publishing. Nevertheless, Jones

(1956) is saying of his type of therapeutic community about this time that there should be 'a single therapeutic goal, namely the adjustment of the individual to social and work conditions outside —*without any ambitious psychotherapeutic programme*' (our italics).

An important issue on which both Main and Jones agree is that the therapeutic community should be given by the wider society in which it operates 'a degree of self determination and freedom of action' (Jones, 1956), 'with no barriers between the hospital and the rest of society' (Main, 1946). Such an ideal remains far from realisation with the outside society and Health Service administration still to a large extent determining the patient's life style once in a hospital, and confirming him in the invalid role by taking away responsibility and denying him many of the rights and privileges of normal members of the community; e.g. no alcohol, no sex and restricted freedom.

The incorporation of therapeutic community ideas

The second stage of therapeutic community development was a period of incorporation of the ideology, in the late 1950s to the mid-1960s. Caine and Smail (1969) summarise the reasons why the therapeutic community took root at this stage as (1) growing dissatisfaction with individual psychotherapy in terms of results and the sheer mass of problems; (2) the emphasis of neo-Freudians such as Fromm and Horney on interpersonal and cultural factors in neurosis; (3) the recognition of the deleterious effects of institutionalisation, (4) the application of social science theories to psychotherapy by Foulkes and others, and (5) the increasing awareness of the importance of social experience in learning and communication processes. Many mental hospitals, starved of other developments in psychiatry while general medicine and surgery had advanced much in the war, avidly took up the therapeutic community idea without any sound conceptualisation of social psychiatry in practice. Open doors, ward meetings and a more liberal regime were all that many mustered in their ignorance, and David Clark (1965) distinguished at this point the therapeutic community approach of those former hospitals and the therapeutic community proper. Of the latter he said they were

(1) in *size* not more than 100 persons, small enough for everyone to be involved with everyone else;

(2) holding regular *meetings of the total community*;
(3) adhering to a *philosophy* that an individual's difficulties were mostly in relation to other people and capable of resolution through discussion;
(4) *analysing the social events* of the unit;
(5) improving the *flow of communications*;
(6) *flattening the authority pyramid*;
(7) providing constant *protected situations* in which patients could try out new ways of coping with difficulties; and
(8) constantly *examining roles and behaviour* in both patients and staff in order to function more effectively.

This decade was a period of implementation of the original ideas but also of discovering the limitations and obstacles to therapeutic community work. Jones originally felt that the method as practised at Belmont was applicable to all psychiatric patients, but research findings at Belmont in the late 1950s by Rapoport and his colleagues who were called in by Maxwell Jones to explore the therapeutic community were initially a setback to the movement. Rapoport (1960) pointed out that the ideology was based on untested convictions and drew attention to many contradictions in practice and theory. The staff held to three basic beliefs, namely

(1) that all activity and interaction in the unit was treatment,
(2) that all treatment was rehabilitation involving both personality reorganisation and adjustment to the social system of the unit and later to the social system pertaining outside; and that,
(3) all patients should be treated alike.

He also draws attention to the specificity of the method and the need for selection of patients. While demonstrating the positive and negative aspects of the therapeutic community dynamics Rapoport identified *four themes* which he saw as shared by the staff:

(1) *democratisation*—each member of the community should share equally in the exercise of power and decision-making without privileged groups or individuals;
(2) *permissiveness*—the community should be able to tolerate the deviant or abnormal behaviour of its members without suppression and at the same time be free to express a reaction to it, the object being to see and understand the real nature of an individual's problems without restricting their expression.

(3) *communalism*—all events in the unit should be a shared experience with the maximum of interrelationship, participation and openness.

(4) *reality confrontation*—an individual's behaviour would constantly be reflected back to him, presenting him with the result, effect or interpretation of his behaviour as it impinged on the various people around him. Thus, there is not the theorising, distancing or hierarchichal presumption of a psychoanalytic interpretation. The confrontation is never 'wrong' or off the mark, as the analyst may be, if one truthfully says 'because *you* behave *thus*, *I* feel or react in *this* way'. This is the basic dynamic of the therapeutic community, which works by the community 'feeding back' to the individual the effects of his behaviour, thus causing him to modify his subsequent behaviour in order to gain a different and more satisfactory response.

The Rapoport study also demonstrated that there could be a conflict of aims for staff and patients in the dual pursuit of treatment (i.e. towards the goal of personality change) as emphasised by medical staff in psychotherapy groups and rehabilitation towards the goal of adjustment to outside circumstances as carried out by non-medical staff in wards and workshops, and this is the point that most subsequent commentators take up. Rapoport suggested that for most patients a planned excursion into one or the other course as appropriate would be more effective, and also, that a grasp of social dynamics and some practice in their manipulation could be harmful to others when maliciously applied outside the treatment context, e.g. by an ex-patient in the patient's family. He further suggested that those with weak ego-structures could be more damaged by exposure to such harsh and powerful techniques without protection or support.

The clarification of therapeutic community practice

In the third developmental stage, from about the mid-1960s, the further analysis and refinement of therapeutic community practice has continued. In the United States, Marshall Edelson (1970) has emerged as a leading theorist in the field. He distinguishes clearly between *psychotherapy*, which he sees as directed at the internal state of the patient, and *sociotherapy*, which he sees as directed at the social situation in which the patient is placed. He keeps the two processes distinct in his therapeutic community practice with different therapists and different occasions for each process, believing that, while the two processes are complementary in the therapeutic community, the intrusion of psychotherapy into a sociotherapy session can be confusing, obstructive or harmful. He sees psychotherapy and sociotherapy as taking the patient in two opposing directions. In sociotherapy, the individual moves from system problems concerned with reality, to goal achievement and thence to a repair of the strains and tensions that have occurred between members of the group in that task. In psychotherapy, the movement is in reverse, from concern with the individual's inner state to orientation in his social environment, and thence to adaptation to it.

The sociotherapist, then, is restricted to identifying and commenting upon the movements and preoccupations of the large community group, and the four common themes are those described by Talcott Parsons (see Chapter 3) as the type of problems that arise in any social system and that the group in any situation will be concerned with for survival. They are:

(1) *adaptation*—to existing situations;
(2) *consummation*—of desired goals;
(3) *integration*—of individuals or sub-groups; and
(4) *motivation*—the expression of group values and maintenance of the group pattern.

The psychotherapy/sociotherapy dichotomy is also expressed in Clark and Yeoman's (1969) study of Frazer House, a therapeutic community in Australia, where separate large group meetings were set aside for *social control* or for *therapy* when the object in the latter was personality change. Clark describes the task of the therapist as identifying the collective foci that may dominate such a free-floating meeting as being problems arising out of situations of (1) threat, (2) loss, (3) gain, or (4) frustration.

In an eminently practical book which describes the establishment of a therapeutic community through successive stages, Margolis (1973) comments that accepting Rapoport's distinction between treatment goals and rehabilitation goals, his ward 'was in the business of rehabilitation—and hoped to get some treatment done as well'. The basic goal was adjustment to the reality of home and work but, complementary to this, to control the patient's deviance, to stabilise his ego-structure and contribute to his ego-growth. Margolis sees the therapeutic community as being able to utilise multiple therapies—individual, group, milieu and the therapy of the community, all essentially interlocked.

The distinction between *psychotherapy* and *sociotherapy* is conceptually helpful, but a skilful blend would seem more in keeping with the original therapeutic community ideology of staff and patients sharing together in the reality of community life in its various phases and commenting, as skills allow, on the events that occur and the roles that are played out rather than distancing the sociotherapist on the edge of the group as expert commentator, which was the position from which the psychotherapist was originally drawn in.

At Henderson *the way* an individual behaves in a situation will be seen as a lead into understanding *why* he reacts in such a way. The social process leads into psychological awareness and personality change is effected through social interaction. For this purpose a complex social system is created within the unit.

(1) *Interaction* is promoted. All matters pertaining to unit life are put routinely to all the members, who are living closely with each other, dependent on each other for emotional and often material support and co-operating (or not) with each other in both large and trivial matters of the day. Interaction is maximised in a way that allows little privacy. In this respect 'all that happens is treatment'—or, as we might now see it, all that happens is worthy of exploration for its effect on the various people concerned. Goffman (1968) has been an outspoken critic of such a practice in therapeutic communities believing that such an intrusion into privacy is unwarranted and that 'looping', as he calls it when information gained in one situation is fed back to the group in another situation or—as he would see it—is used against the patient, is unjustifiable.

In the therapeutic community it should be made clear at the outset and repeated that the method relies upon all happenings and communications being brought into the open because they are pertinent to the complex task of understanding behaviour that has often thwarted other treatment approaches already. This must be the *contract* under which patients enter therapeutic community treatment. The intensive interaction between individuals in this setting has been described by a patient as 'like real life speeded up—you meet in twenty-four hours situations you wouldn't meet in twenty-four days outside!'

(2) *Exploration* of observed behaviour is then essential to the understanding of it. Group meetings provide the richest source of feed-back from different viewpoints, and groups with different structures, compositions, settings and overt tasks add to the opportunities for getting a balanced feed-back overall. The daily large group meeting is the keystone of the therapeutic community. It provides for social control but also for identification with the common purpose. Regressive and exaggerated emotional response is a feature of the large group (see chapter 6), but it is also the setting in which goals formulated by the group can be achieved by co-operative functioning. The large group has power and can see the result of using that power in a very short time. It has strength and can give strength to its members, facing and overcoming very real anxieties. Small group meetings, which follow more classically on the group-analytic model, allow for deeper reflection on the immediate experiences of the living situation and provide the opportunity for relating present experience to past experience. Activity groups of various kinds make up the patient's day. These will be task-orientated work groups to keep the practical aspects of the living situation in working order, administrative groups dealing with the admission of patients, catering, social events and future planning, or crisis meetings of part or all of the community should they be required, and role-playing, encounter and similar experiential groups. Throughout all the groups and activities runs the 'contract' of treatment, namely that all that occurs should be examined for what it might disclose of an individual's pattern of behaviour.

(3) *Experimentation* with new modes of behaviour must then follow if old behaviour, having occurred and been examined, is to be replaced. At Henderson a somewhat ritualistic and repetitive cycle of events provides the structure within which this can occur. All patients will be elected by their fellows into one or other of the jobs within the community. Thus, wards and workshops have their representatives, meetings their chairmen and certain specialised roles; for example, the selection team interviewing prospective patients, or social work assistants reserved for more experienced patients. Each month the jobs are reallocated by the group according to observed treatment needs rather than abilities. Thus, a

phobic patient who would sit by the door is appointed the 'teller', whereby he has to face the space in the middle of the room to count votes. In an examination of the formal roles and changes in behaviour that might occur during their tenure, Manor (1977) divided the jobs into three categories and questioned staff as to the ideal behaviour for such a post-holder and how far a particular individual was seen to approach the ideal in his tenure of office. His findings were as follows.

(a) The *administrative* jobs, such as chairman of the community, although much sought after on a prestige basis, produced little personality change. People who were manipulative and controlling on the outside tended to take these jobs and no new behaviour emerged.

(b) The *service* jobs, such as cooks or storemen, were frequently handed out on the grounds that it would 'do you good to serve others', but were so beset by negative sanctions, complaints and hustle that, if anything, antagonistic and deviant behaviour was only re-entrenched.

(c) The *creative* posts, such as ward representative, workshop leader or social work assistant, where little negative sanction was evident but a great deal of positive reward was bestowed on the individual, either overtly, if he accomplished a task for the community, or less publicly when he was instrumental in assisting a fellow patient, provided most scope for change in a positive direction.

Experiences in the therapeutic community

The individual in a therapeutic community passes through a series of complicated involvements, of which staff must be aware, if they are to act with discernment.

The *large group*, favoured in the staff ideology of a therapeutic community, is usually seen by patients as a tense, threatening, punitive or confusing meeting and least orientated to treatment. Staff will adhere to the ideological tenet when questioned, but in practice many of them share the view of the patients. Manning (1976), in an investigation of values and practice in the therapeutic community, illustrated how many of the staff, like the patients, prefer to work in the areas where psychotherapy is practised rather

117

than in the sociotherapeutic arena although professing the opposite. The large group can be excited, regressive and at times frightening, as it provokes primitive behaviour in the competition for recognition and confirmation of one's existence. Quieter members go to the wall and literally hide in the dark corners, but for some passive, withdrawn and seemingly under-stimulated individuals the excitement engendered may provide the very stimulation they lack in normal interaction and an explosive outburst from someone else finds them warming, as it were, at the flames. The danger is that they actively provoke disorder in others in order to achieve this effect. The general anonymity of the community meeting can similarly produce contradictory results. On the one hand, remarks addressed generally to the centre of the room are not as anxiety-laden as if made face-to-face with an individual; but on the other hand, when a remark is generally made and no one responds or even seems to hear, the feeling of isolation, alienation or even non-existence can be enhanced. For some with particular anxieties about individual relationships the general relationship with the amorphous large group is a first and less loaded step towards personal relationships, whereas for others the seeming denial of a personal and private relationship in the community is a frightening and anxiety-raising experience. It is for the skilled therapist to be aware of the various implications for different individuals. Transference relationships in the therapeutic community are an important source of treatment and quickly develop despite the superficial proclamation that 'we are all equal'. Such relationships must not be diminished or dismissed. They are intense because old emotional experiences are rapidly reawakened in the highly charged atmosphere with its multiple opportunities for transferred relationships to parent figures, sibling substitutes, old friends, the real or fantasised family or society at large. Staff members are particularly cast in this role, primarily because of the roles that they are perceived to occupy and second because of their real personalities. Patients, too, may be seen as envied or favoured siblings. The myth that 'we are all equal' was one of many misconceptions about the therapeutic community that Morrice (1972) drew attention to; in the matter of transference relationship, this is quite evident, and a valuable treatment opportunity must not be cast aside in the pursuit of a spurious equality. In the large group the appropriate interjection from the relevant transference figure makes a meaningful point, whereas the same remark from another can be disregarded. This is particularly so in the questions of 'law and order' when a response from the leader is invested with great authority and provides the security and control that the rule-breaker is often seeking by his agitated acting-out.

The course through the therapeutic community follows a predictable path. New members, however enthusiastically they sought admission, very quickly settle down into the pattern of behaviour with which they are familiar and feel safe. The community provides no diversionary 'hospital treatment' procedures with which they can become occupied and the customary interpersonal behaviour in the living situation, for which the new patient has probably been referred for treatment, soon appears. He makes the situation a 'viable' one, in the terminology of Whitaker and Lieberman (1965), and one in which he can survive by his accustomed defensive ploys, acting-out avoidance of emotional stress and general manipulation of others to his needs. The early weeks are most difficult for the rest of the community, who must tolerate this but at the same time gently and supportively confront and attempt to curtail it. The new patient reaches a stage in a matter of two or three weeks when either it is put to him bluntly that he must change or else he realises himself that in order to stay he has to alter. At this point some 20 to 30 per cent will leave, which is comparable with drop-outs from other psychotherapy and for the same reasons. A few experience a 'flight into health', others begin to change, and family or marital partners persuade them to leave because the *status quo* of that relationship is about to alter. Most will leave because they see the commitment to treatment to be too much for them, the way ahead arduous and no obviously dramatic changes likely to occur. Defences are forcefully held on to and when manipulations of the new environment fail they summarily depart. For those who remain there then follows a quick assumption of a *positive transference* to the unit that seems to promise so much. They incorporate all the ritual, take on the jobs enthusiastically and praise the unit to outsiders. Under personal stress, however, they revert to acting-out behaviour to avoid a feeling response. Gradually relationships are made and in a situation of more security emotional feelings are experienced instead of avoided. Acting-out behaviour diminishes but in two to three months the individual will often complain that he is worse than on admission—depressed, hopeless, inadequate and facing an empty or frightening future. Now comes a stage of *negative* transference to the unit, which he feels has given him nothing but hurt. At the same time however this feeling person is often most active in helping newcomers. Gradually the good and the bad are brought into perspective, reality is substituted for fantasy and a more balanced personality emerges.*

Leaving the community is a difficult time and the transition to the unchanged world outside with the new patterns of behaviour can be an anxious period. One follow-up study at Henderson illustrated that relapse in the early weeks after leaving was not uncommon—but was not a portent of further lapses when follow-up was extended over some years (Copas and Whiteley, 1976). The relapses were often trivial incidents, almost a tentative testing-out of reality. One ex-patient said after a few weeks, 'I'm just the same —fighting the cops, handcuffed, thinking I'm King Kong—*but I know what I'm doing*, now. That's the difference.' With time, the testing-out period passes and insight leads to a more settled behaviour.

At different stages in the treatment process different points of emphasis can be made. Matza (1969), in his description of 'becoming deviant', has described the social processes by which a behavioural pattern is learned. The situation for the emotionally disturbed patient is analagous. A deviant pattern of interaction with his fellows has been set up and in treatment we seek to replace this

---

*For example, an ex-patient writes: 'I find that I have to consider my wife and children now. Which I never gave a thought of before I went to Henderson. I told you in my last letter that as I did not feel like a Robot anymore I was finding it difficult handling feelings. Well I find it a lot better and easier now. In fact it's quite nice. Especially towards my family. I find that I really think ahead now instead of doing things impulsively. It's very difficult to explain to you what I mean. As nearly all the things I feel now are new to me. I think what has happened to me is that when I was at Henderson I lived my life again. But whilst I was living it again I was taught right from wrong also I was feeling things (emotions etc) also I was getting feelings from the staff to share. Also I was getting rid of my aggression. But you see the great thing for me at Henderson was that the staff told "truly" how they felt towards you and your behaviour. But still wanted to help and understand you. But help you to understand yourself at the same time. To put it in a nutshell to me I grew up at Henderson with good foster parents. "Staff." '

through a relearning process. The social forces that Matza describes in the case of acquiring a deviant image can be identified in the relearning process.

(1) *affinity*—whereby the individual cleaves to, and is most influenced by, those with whom he has things in common. In the early days of treatment staff should stand back and let the peer-group get to grips with the newcomer, his expectations, anxieties, and currently held patterns of behaviour. The newcomer will be trying to re-assert the accustomed patterns (making the situation *viable*) and in the hospital situation, particularly, trying to invoke the doctor and patient interaction which, if he succeeds, will eradicate any therapeutic community influence. At Henderson an experienced patient acts as co-therapist in the introductory group for new patients. As the new patients are introduced, at weekly intervals over a period of three weeks, even last week's admissions are soon bringing an influence to bear on this week's newcomers.

(2) *affiliation*—the need to join and be accepted and recognised by an established group with a corporate identity. The jargon, customs, rules and rituals of the therapeutic community provide the trappings of the 'club' into which the newcomer is accepted provided he takes them on. For this reason it is important for staff to go along with the culture and not dismiss it as unsophisticated. The rituals have a purpose in providing the matrix within which relationships and associations can be made.

(3) *signification*—the recognition by society that the individual can be expected to act in a certain way. He is 'labelled', and all subsequent behaviour is tagged with the label earlier applied. In treatment the experimentation with new roles and different behaviour only succeeds if others can discard the old label and acknowledge, and indeed underline, the new behaviour when it emerges, giving it and the individual a new signification or label.

Fluctuations in group life occur in the therapeutic community as in the outside society. Rapoport (1960) drew attention to the cycles of organisation and disorganisation in the therapeutic community, the search for leaders with particular attributes (supportive, creative, authoritarian, punitive, etc.) in one phase and for those with other attributes at another time. For staff, who will live and work through several such cycles even in a twelve-month period, some awareness of the dynamics is necessary so that they, at least, can retain a hold on reality and at some times facilitate the emergence of the appropriate behaviour or leader while at other times withdraw and allow the group to flourish unaided and without interference.

Results from therapeutic communities

Evaluating the effectiveness of the therapeutic community in terms of outcome is comparable to asking—does *progressive education* work? While certain results have been published (Whiteley, 1970; Copas and Whiteley, 1976; Clark and Yeomans, 1969; Myers and Clark, 1972; Craft *et al.*, 1964; Miles, 1969a, b; Cornish and Clarke, 1975), and in some cases controlled trials carried out, the review by Clarke and Cornish (1972) of the problems of institutional research and the particular complexities of research into the therapeutic community outline the hazards of drawing conclusions from this type of enquiry.

The simple, drug trial, method with a quick response of cured or not cured cannot be applied to a treatment which is long-term, open to innumerable outside influences and where, in any case, the objective outcome criteria are vague. A flight into process studies, which try to pin-point what particular aspect of the treatment affects which particular symptoms or personality variables, and in what particular way, is one consequence, but for true evaluation both *outcome* and *process* studies must be conducted.

An early controlled trial of a therapeutic community was Craft's study (Craft *et al.*, 1964) of psychopaths at Balderton. The groups were randomly assigned to therapeutic community and authoritarian regimes and at follow-up it was found that the latter group was more successful in terms of fewer reconvictions or fewer readmissions to institutions. However, process factors must be taken into account. These were adolescent offenders of low intelligence, compulsorily detained for treatment; and it could be inferred that the appropriate treatment approach to this particular problem boy would be a more directive and supportively controlling one, rather than investing him with a responsibility that he was unable to carry. Miles (1969a), in a similar controlled study of subnormal psychopathic offenders, measured the development of interpersonal relationships and found that the therapeutic community increased the ability for this, whereas the traditional treatment methods did not. In a further study Miles (1969b) went on to show that attitudes of hostility to authority were changed in a positive way in the therapeutic community group and unchanged in the traditionally treated group.

Two studies at Henderson, by Whiteley (1970) and Copas and Whiteley (1976), have shown improvement in the behaviour of psychopaths (of normal intelligence and voluntary patients) but with no control group for comparison. The first study (1970) reported that 40 per cent had no further social relapse in the follow-up period of two to three years, in terms of reconviction or re-admission to hospital. The study showed that those who responded to the particular, peer-group, regime of Henderson, with its admixture of sociotherapy and psychotherapy, as already outlined, were those who could be regarded as *'creative'* personalities with some evidence of ability to succeed at school, work or in marriage and able to express themselves in a feeling way. Those who failed were the more 'inadequate', institutionalised, personalities dependent on the social or penal services and with little achievement in the school, work or interpersonal fields. The second study (Copas and Whiteley, 1976) showed that 47 per cent were successful, according to the same criteria, over the three-year period while 40 per cent continued free of relapse over a five-to-six-year period. From these two studies it was possible to produce and validate a predictive equation, the factors weighted being length of time in work, marital history, educational achievement, criminality and psychiatric history. It is suggested that these are all factors that bear some relevance to creative, dynamic, emotional life and hence would be appropriately met by therapeutic community treatment.

A not dissimilar picture emerges from studies of schizophrenics treated in the therapeutic community. Letemendia *et al.* (1967), in a country mental hospital at Oxford, were able randomly to assign the chronic schizophrenic population to a therapeutic community programme or to a traditionally run mental hospital programme, when the hospital was originally thus divided. At follow-up after three years they were unable to show any difference in the two groups.

Myers and Clark (1972), at Cambridge, reported that disturbed schizophrenics responded better to the therapeutic community ward than to the orthodox ward used as a control and argue that it is the disturbed psychotics, 'still struggling with their fate and reacting against their institutional environment', who are the ones able to benefit from feed-back from the therapeutic community whereas the overall study of Letemendia must have included all types of schizophrenics.

This again illustrates the difficulty of generalising from overall studies of a loose diagnostic group or a total population. In the schizophrenic study of Letemendia, as in the Henderson study or the Cornish and Clarke (1975) study of approved school boys, some types respond well, some types respond badly and some are unaffected. Overall, the results even out and show 'no change', and therefore identification of the interactive processes becomes vitally important.

Before leaving the schizophrenic group further reference to another study by Miles (1972) can be made. In this, chronic schizophrenics treated in a therapeutic community workshop were shown to increase the extent of their interpersonal relationships when compared with a control group.

Caine and Smail (1969) found psychotics and personality disorder patients less likely to respond to a therapeutic community, however. They compared neurotics treated in a five-day week residential unit run on rather psychotherapeutic community lines with similar patients in mental hospitals and a neurosis unit. They showed that the patients in the therapeutic community unit changed significantly in both symptoms and personality measures when compared with the control group and the changes were sustained four to five years later. An earlier paper by Martin and Caine (1963) demonstrated beneficial changes in personality in chronic neurotics as a result of therapeutic community treatment.

A final research report by Clark (1967) indicated that patient improvement in the therapeutic community at Frazer House was related to the extent of his participation, verbally and physically, in the activities and affairs of the unit.

The application of the therapeutic community

Maxwell Jones has more recently commented that there is no one model for a therapeutic community. Moos (1974) gives four examples of differently organised therapeutic communities, each claiming some success for its method with a particular type of patient. He cites, first, the original Maxwell Jones (1953) model with its emphasis on involvement, peer group support, autonomy and independence, with staff control played down. This was aimed in the main at young adults with personality disorders.

Fairweather (1964) constructed problem–orientated task groups to provide chronic patients, prior to discharge, with experience in more active roles than had been open to them in the heavily dependent hospital situation. The patients proceeded in stages of increasing responsibility with considerable patient involvement in the administration and evaluation. At follow-up, those involved in the programme were more likely to be actively engaged outside the hospital than patients treated in the traditional way. Sanders *et al.* (1967) organised three socio-environmental programmes with (1) minimal structure but some opportunities for interaction; (2) more structured interactional groups for discussions and co-operative tasks and (3) a maximally structured programme with large and small group meetings, patient government and high interaction. The response was that the older and more chronic patients (who were unaffected by a traditional ward programme running as a control) responded better to the highly structured programme and this improvement was sustained in subsequent community adjustment. The younger patients and those with a shorter duration of illness responded less well to these socio-environmental treatment programmes, seeming disturbed by the interpersonal intimacy demanded. Coleman (1971) designed a treatment programme for disturbed delinquents who had responded poorly to a regular ward routine. A token economy system was employed but non-directive group therapy had little impact in changing behaviour, whereas practical instructional periods concerned with social skills and interests provoked a positive shift in attitudes to work and peer relationships.

One of the critical findings of Rapoport's (1960) study of the Maxwell Jones's unit was that carry-over of improved behaviour learned in the unit to the outside did not always occur, and this was attributed to the fact that the staff at that time failed to appreciate that patients were largely from lower socio-economic groups qualified only for unskilled and semi-skilled work positions and accustomed to working under supervision. Returning to similar conditions outside, their newly acquired behaviour was inappropriate. Similarly, the Fairweather study had quite a high readmission rate despite some successes, again suggesting that a carry-over of in-treatment progress did not always occur. This was attributed to the fact that a pattern of group interaction and support had been learned but on the outside the ex-patient had to function as an individual. Channelled into group homes rather than into the general community, their overall functioning improved as the newly acquired group support behaviour could be utilised.

The present Henderson experience already referred to illustrates the different responses of different personality types to the current programme.

Out of these studies the points that emerge are that there is an interaction between the particular treatment programme and the different personality types involved and that the final treatment outcome is effected by the environment to which the patient is returned. Also, the American version of the therapeutic community tends more towards the structured socio-therapeutic programme, even overtly behaviourist in some situations, than does the English one with its bias towards psychotherapy.

Some selection of patients for any one specific therapeutic community programme therefore seems advisable, and the idea of having a mix of different personality types and problems, as in a microcosm of the outside world, is more likely to lead to weakening of the group ethos and splintering of the treatment process in an attempt to meet the varied needs of the various patient types, leading to conflict and confusion.

Staff reactions to the therapeutic community

The staff in a therapeutic community are exposed to and experience the same sociodynamic and psychodynamic forces as do the patients if they are positively and actively involved. Acting-out behaviour occurs at a less pathological level than in the patient group, but lateness, failure to communicate information and rejection of the staff values in favour of deviant patient values at times occur. Staff groups both large and small with administrative and interpersonal tasks and also groups with intra-personal objectives are necessary, not only as a corrective experience for staff under stress but also as a learning experience. For efficient running of the unit an individual's behaviour must be monitored by the peer group and, just as for patients, this should be a 'contract' of participation in the staff of a therapeutic community. Zeitlyn (1975), among others, has taken the therapeutic community staff to task for the time spent in self-examination, but the parallels that run between preoccupations and crises in the staff group and similar ones in the patient group are indicative of the shared stresses that encompass a therapeutic community and staff resolution of their problems can lead the way into facilitation of patient resolution of the problem as seen in that arena.

Under personal stress, a Henderson investigation showed, the staff member retreats into the formalised role that he knows best (Whiteley and Zlatic, 1972). The doctor begins to give medical opinions, for instance, which the non-medical cannot challenge. All staff felt more worthwhile and productive when in the formalised role of their profession, despite the professed allegiance to 'role-blurring', than in the more open and personally vulnerable area of interaction as a genuine member of the community.

Nevertheless, the staff member in a therapeutic community has attitudes to treatment different from his colleagues in traditional treatment settings. Caine and Smail (1966) showed by an Attitudes Questionnaire that the therapeutic community doctor, in comparison with his non-therapeutic community colleague, would be likely to be more permissive and less controlling, more intent on sharing the role of therapist, preferring a personal to a professional approach and psychological to physical treatments, rejecting the role of individual therapist, aiming treatment at personality change as much as at symptom relief and looking on treatment as disturbing rather than palliative. He would appear not to distinguish between psychotic and neurotic patients quite as sharply as the more traditionally orientated psychiatrist.

6   The large group

The large group is an integral part of therapeutic community practice and indeed is the major factor that distinguishes the therapeutic community process from other hospital treatment programmes. Daily, formalised large group meetings take place in a therapeutic community. They have a special relationship to the other activities of the day and it could well be said that the twenty-four hours of the therapeutic community is one kind of continuous large group. Interest in the large group itself has been revived by some members of the Institute of Group Analysis in the 1970s and de Maré (1972) is one who suggests it as a possible approach to treatment in its own right. 'The problem for the member of the small group is how to feel spontaneously,' he comments, 'whereas for the large group it is primarily how to think.' While there is an enormous flow of information in the large group,

> intelligence is only too easily blocked by the energy flow;
> intelligence succumbs to coercion; the loud mouth silences
> the still voice of intuition; affiliative communication 'on the
> level' gives way to hierarchical non-communication; leading
> ideas and trends give way to the pressures and transferences
> of personality and leadership.

The compulsion to repeat the family interrelationships in the large group is enormous, he goes on, but the result in the large group is a structure neither gratifying nor realistic. The members then have to reshape this model and de Maré believes that the capacity for change in the large group is immense. Projected feelings and role-playing relationships are so tangible and so much more amplified and manifest than in the small group and what has to be maintained, he says, is an openness for action and interaction between the self-system of the individual and the social system of the large group.

Looking at the large group situation we see that large groups are both natural and contrived.

The *natural* large groups that occur are open to the group-dynamic forces described by Lewin (1951) and others (see chapter 3), and evidence the typical patterns of behaviour and interaction that Freud (1921) and his predecessors had described. Such natural large groups occur in colleges, industry, clubs, political parties, government, nations, etc. The *contrived* large groups are either for *treatment* or *study* purposes. The treatment groups are a part of a therapeutic community approach when they exhibit a particular relationship to the whole or are treatment procedures in their own right as de Maré promulgates. The large group as a unit for the study of interpersonal and intrapersonal processes has been fostered by the psychoanalytic, the sociological and the experiential schools.

Group dynamics research into the variable of size provides evidence that size limits the type and frequency of possible communications in a group. Members must deal with a more complicated range of relationships with less time and fewer resources. Turquet (1974a), for example, notes that sixteen chess pieces are about the limit that a person can keep in mind at one time, and strictly cognitive problems seem to arise in groups of over six or seven when it becomes necessary to think in terms of sub-groups, classes or stereotypes. The formula $X = \frac{1}{2}(3^n - 2^{n+1} + 1)$ gives some idea of the number of potential relationships between individuals, between sub-groups and between individuals and sub-groups where n is the number of members. In a family of six there are 301 such relationships (Hare, 1962). The development of leadership in larger groups reduces this cognitive and emotional complexity by substituting a series of pair relationships between each member and the leader. The need for leadership also arises from the increasing problems of co-ordination that size entails. While it is more difficult to achieve consensus as size increases, large groups potentially offer more judgements, ideas, skills and power. These advantages, however, may reach a limit as difficulty in co-ordination brings diminishing returns (Hare, 1962).

Contrived groups; the large group in treatment

(a) *As part of the therapeutic community* the large group has a multiple function. It is the common meeting ground, where faith in the treatment process is daily affirmed; it is the communications centre, the control agent and a teaching situation. It also provokes issues for discussion and primes emotional feelings in a heightened atmosphere of tension and excitement, so that feelings are expressed in an explosive, uncontrolled and often exaggerated way. In association with small group therapy, where such issues can be examined in a safe and more rational way, the large group experience leads into otherwise unplumbed waters, but wise and sensitive leadership is necessary lest the large group phenomena run away with the situation or unscrupulous members of the group simply stir the action for excitement's sake. When to promote anxiety and when to hold back, for instance, are issues about which the staff must be clear. A particularly troublesome patient may have stormed out of the meeting yet again, thus contravening rule so-and-so. 'Bring him back,' shouts the group, 'he's discharged if he isn't back in 5 minutes when the group ends.' The posse of strong arm men race for the door and need to be told, 'Hold it—what are we doing? If you force him back now there'll be a fight—and then another discharge vote. He's going to miss 5 minutes of the group. Perhaps if we leave him to cool down and whoever can best talk to him can make sure he goes to the small group. . . .'

The place of the large group in the mental hospital has been referred to by Jones and Hollingsworth (1963b), who see it as reducing disturbances in the ward by resolving misunderstandings and interpersonal conflicts but who particularly stress the learning opportunity it affords the staff. Marohn (1967) echoes this purpose in describing the large group meeting in a correctional establishment for youths. The primary purpose of unit meetings was to intervene with a proven therapeutic technique into the inmate-officer interaction world before a chain of mutual mistrust–acting-out–punishment and exile was established. Furedi et al. (1974) state that the direct intention of the ward community is the regulation of behaviour and the correction of behaviour with the help of rules made in common. Thus, social control and 'treatment' through behaviour modification features high in the expressed purposes of the large group meeting in a therapeutic community.

Although Edelson (1970) appears to take the therapeutic purpose further by seeing the large group as engaged in a task of understanding social processes and resolving social conflict situations and learning through this experience, insight into interpersonal problems is not set as a primary target by many of those who have described the large group in this setting. The introduction of more psychotherapeutic techniques and theories into the large group is possible, however. Springmann (1970) enthusiastically depends upon a wholly psychoanalytic approach. Kreeger (1974) believes that psychotherapy in the large group is possible given skilled leadership, and Pines (1974) describes the large meeting as a situation in which a relevant informational network can be developed and personally significant issues presented and transacted. He utilised the daily large group as an introductory exercise and an adjunct to the small group psychotherapy which would follow and be enhanced by the earlier interpersonal activity.

Curry (1967), however, in a critical examination of the literature pertaining to large groups, was of the opinion that psychotherapy in the large group did not take place and that what behavioural modification or social control appeared to take place was questionable because of the capacity of the individual to assume an apparent conformity to the group while resisting any actual internal change of behaviour.

The daily large group meeting is the keystone of a therapeutic community. Without it the patients would merely wait for their 'treatment session' with the group therapist, occupying one-and-a-half hours each day, and 'the other 23 (or $22\frac{1}{2}$) hours' of the patient's day that Stanton and Schwartz (1954) refer to would be lost. The community meeting draws together the therapeutic strands, but exactly how it should be run or on what theoretical model it should be based is in considerable doubt. Much more exploratory research is required about the precise nature of the community meeting. The only theory that does seem agreed from the literature is that a very skilled and perceptive leadership is required, not necessarily by one therapist but through an informed staff team united in effort and in ideological approach, perhaps utilising a sensitive blend of sociotherapy and psychotherapy.

(b) *The large group as an entity* is described in detail in a book edited by Kreeger (1974) which examines various large group situations. In these chapters as well as in other papers on the large group, there is a remarkable consensus of agreement on observed large group behaviour. Again, much of this simply reiterates the nineteenth-century writings of Le Bon (1895), but Kreeger pinpoints the common desire of the large group to split into subgroups rather than work through a stress situation; the psychotic mechanisms which seem to be released in a large group in a way that parallels the infant's primitive perception of reality; the threat to identity and emergence of paranoid anxieties; manic flight and sexual fantasy as a defence against deeper depressive preoccupations. The leadership position is stressed. Large groups tend to dependency reactions, battles for leadership emerge and the leadership role is exacting and responsible, perhaps in a way that small group leadership in its less obtrusive pattern is less so.

Main (1974) more deeply explores some of the psychodynamic mechanisms of the large group that give rise to the phenomena described. He sees in particular that the large group affords massive projection opportunities, so that the individual on the one hand is projecting out on to the many others his unwanted parts while he (and others) are the subjects of the projections of other group members. Thus, individuals become depleted and non-beings, as it were. Anonymity prevails. The individual members feel valueless and the group is endowed with everything. Thus, people feel unable to contribute unless they can formulate some great 'Nobel-prize' statement, whereas others invested with idealised projections respond in a *prima donna* way. The feeling that one cannot compete or participate at such a high level leads members to dismiss invitations to take part and to fear the envy of others, should they have the courage to take on a role in the group.

The group often begins in an awkward and hesitant way with prolonged silences, and after the group has concluded (and Main and others comment on how the group is only too glad to reach its end) members sort into twos and threes of familiar friendly bodies to break into animated and relieved talk in order to 'get back their own identity'. The staff after-group meeting is but an institutionalised and formal way of doing this. In the small group it is easier to keep contact with people; there are fewer projections flying around and people retain a hold on themselves, feel capable of questioning attitudes or behaviour attributed to them and rejecting or modifying it, with the help of others. In the large group you are on your own, which Turquet (1974b) also points out. The 'singleton', as he describes the individual member, finds it difficult to establish contact and relationships in the large group and feels a threat to his identity.

Directing his attention to the therapeutic aspect of the large group, Main pleads caution. Large groups are rarely united in one direction and therefore group interpretations are seldom valid and often no more than projections themselves, revealing more of the unconscious beliefs of the one who offers them. He advises that interventions should be more in the nature of personal statements to emphasise the reality of the situation, the feelings and the identity of the group members.

However, Springmann (1974) is one who has developed the idea of *psychotherapy in the large group*.

Large meetings (fifty patients) of patients of mixed diagnoses were originally brought together weekly, with their attendant staff and the group leader, in an attempt to 'regulate the atmosphere' in which treatment could proceed. When the psychotherapeutic potential was realised the objective of the group was altered in that direction. Springmann describes both individual and group responses to the free interaction in an unstructured and undefined framework and therapist responses to both. He appreciates the intensity of feeling and the need for therapist intervention when other patients can 'rip apart' the defences of one individual but, equally, the way in which the encouragement and stimulus of the group can lead one individual on into deep excursions into past memories, fantasy and perceptions, and can moderate present feeling and reaction in a way that the individual therapist may be powerless to do. The patient will 'listen to the voice of the mass' on what is reasonable or acceptable but may reject an individual therapist's opinion on the same issue. The large group dilutes the transference and thus allows some child–parent feelings to be expressed freely. The mass is a challenge to the withdrawn patient to show himself and register his being but at the same time is anonymous enough for him to do so without fear of repercussion. Springmann (1974) remarks on the development of a group maturation and group memory as mechanisms and ways of behaviour, and information on past incidents is woven into the culture and carried from generation to generation so that 'the group' comes to act in a more constructive way than a haphazardly assembled crowd.

Springmann also comments on the way both the Bion (1961) basic assumptions can be discerned in the large group and, in particular, how Ezriel's (1959) object-relationship theory can be identified. Thus he describes an incident where another therapist took Springmann unannounced into a large group. The group largely indulged in complaining about the behaviour of authority figures (father, landlord, etc.) elsewhere who intruded upon their privacy, yet they dare not protest for fear of rejection or eviction. An object–relations analysis and interpretation would have related the past reflections to the present situation. In his development of psychotherapy in the large group Springmann leans towards a leader-centred therapy in which transference to the leader is pre-eminent.

(c) *The large group as a medium for sociotherapy*, i.e. the exploration of the interpersonal dynamics and interactions between people in their present social situation (e.g. patients living together in a hospital ward), is dealt with in more detail in chapter 5, but can be briefly summarised here. Edelson (1970) is the advocate of large group therapy wherein the sociotherapist (who is a different person from the psychotherapist, who will be treating the patients concerned in the large group in separate individual or group-analytic sessions) directs his attention to the social dynamics of the group alone and excludes any psychotherapeutic interventions. Thus he concentrates on the types of group movements and mechanisms described by Parsons (see chapter 3), making explicit and facilitating the resolution of conflicts around the group drives towards

(1) adaptation;
(2) integration;
(3) consummation; and
(4) motivation.

Edelson uses the large group to explore the social determinants of behaviour rather than the intra-psychic and goes so far as to say that psychotherapeutic interventions in what is basically a social conflict situation are obstructive to the task in hand.

However a *combination of sociotherapy and psychotherapy* as seems appropriate to the immediate situation is yet a third method of large group work. Schiff and Glassman (1969), in a paper that is both theoretical and practical, compare the Edelson (sociotherapeutic) approach with what they term the Maxwell Jones (sociotherapy and psychotherapy admixture) method, which again is dealt with more fully in chapter 5. They comment that the large group therapist must modify his style from the accustomed small group (psychotherapy) approach and be aware of certain large group phenomena. They emphasise that, in the large group, sub-groups and cliques and sub-systems of behaviour form. There is a wealth of information coming in and a variety of behavioural patterns may co-exist. The group can be overwhelmed by this output and become unable to function or find direction frequently expressing despair and hopelessness. Rice (1951) has pointed out that as size increases in industrial settings the emotional tone fluctuates from aggression to dependency and back again. So in large groups, say Schiff and Glassman, there is more dependency on the leader and more intense affective orderings. With fewer opportunities to be heard there can be a breakdown of communication between members; a feeling of isolation can be enhanced; in order to be seen and heard the members resort to exaggerated behaviour; extremes of activity and control or passivity and submissiveness are seen. Indeed, the feeling of insignificance or nonexistence can be enhanced when remarks are made not person-to-person but into the body of the room, and when a remark is made and not one of fifty people present responds! Schiff and Glassman suggest four goals for the therapist: (1) *selection of topics* (not necessarily directly but perhaps by leading in), to avert the dependency–aggression cycle; (2) *maintaining the safe group-climate*, so that exaggerated hostility, scapegoating, suppression or dominance by one sub-group is eliminated; (3) *gate-keeping*, by which is meant inviting more silent members to involve themselves in the problem-solving, limiting monopolisation and sharing out the topics in such a way that more people can be involved; and (4) *modelling* of patients on their therapists' behaviour, which occurs more intensively in the large group. In the small group there are greater affectional ties between members and mutual responsiveness and the therapist can be allowed to act in a largely passive way, which is quite the opposite of how he wants the patients to behave. In the large group the greater distance between members and the less intense affectional ties direct more attention to the leader. Cues are taken from his behaviour, therefore he must now operate in a less traditionally 'psychoanalytic' way and be a more active leader, whom the members can imitate and thus enhance their own interpersonal functioning.

The more seemingly ill-defined, but intentionally more open, sociotherapy–psychotherapy see-saw of large group interaction, as utilised by Schiff and Glassman and ourselves at Henderson, can none the less have moments of great 'psychotherapeutic' interchange. For one thing, the *group focal conflict* (Whitaker and Lieberman, 1965) processes seem particularly applicable to large group dynamics but require the perceptive ear and action of a skilled staff team to keep the flow in the required direction. Thus, in a group described in detail and transcript elsewhere (Whiteley, *et al.*, 1972), a Henderson large group assembled to review the situation in the hospital workshops.

Both staff and patients expressed their concern that the work tasks were not being carried out (the *disturbing motive*). Ideas such as keeping a register were floated (*restrictive solutions*). Suggestions that we could plan work ahead for only a week at a time so that we can see results (*enabling solutions*) are ignored, and more ideas such as making a list of the jobs to be done (*restrictive solutions*) are floated. People return to the idea of just planning one job at a time and achieving that (the *enabling solution*), but dither backwards and forwards until, under some pressure from the staff group, they begin to say *why they cannot commit themselves* to a task. There is a fear that present agreement will mean commitment 'for ever and ever'; another feels that he will not be able to get involved in the group and will have to 'float off', and a third that the job will never be done to his satisfaction and he will either have to seek control or run away from it (these are the *reactive fears*). With these anxieties out in the open and related to real-life experiences on the outside, the group begins to get together to plan its work as a treatment exercise and is keen to make a start, when some of the staff members in the workshop seem to be throwing up blocks by saying that certain materials needed cannot be got ready in time. It is suggested in a later staff meeting that they were seeing themselves superseded by the patient group and losing their control over the latter. The patient group press on with their plans but the *reactive fears* return or are expressed again in view of the blocks put up by the staff members. Another patient finally rescues the day by suggesting another task which can be done by the same group in a brief exercise and without needing the materials that the staff members had been doubtful about providing (*enabling solution*). A different group however took a more classically psychoanalytic direction. It assembled light-heartedly enough with one of the male patients playing with a child's doll like a ventriloquist as the members assembled. The doll was particularly made to greet myself as I came in. The doll-player had also resigned from the position of authority in the community because he could not reconcile the expectation of the community, that he should control or discipline people, with his own fears that his feelings could get out of hand and he would be excessively punitive or misjudge a situation. The two chairmen of the community, Jim and Jean, continued to remark on the irresponsibility of some patients who made impossible demands and the need to organise the breakfast rotas properly. Silences became longer. An announcement was made that, as the hospital catering officer was away, special food wanted for a party could not be obtained. There was even a garbled message that no food at all was to be sent to us from the kitchen on that night. One of the chairmen, Jim, said after a long silence that he felt isolated.

'Why don't you play with us', said Bill quite seriously, although everyone laughed. He meant that Jim did not take part in games like chess, Monopoly, cards, etc., with the others. There was some defensive intellectualisation by Jim and further silence.

'I really think you ought to play with us', repeated Bill, to more laughter. Jean thought Jim was trying to stir up material for a discussion by saying he was isolated. Jim said, 'let's talk about someone else, then', and the possibility of buying food for the party was raised. I asked Jim what the 'come and play with us' suggestion stirred up in him.

'I don't want to play any more', he answered. The patients who were missing group sessions were then accused of playing games.

'So are you, then', came retorts in a childish way. 'I'd like to play with *you* about midnight', said introverted and inhibited Bob to Mary, as everyone giggled.

The mood shifted to the way people irritated and annoyed others and Jim re-entered the group to ask why Mona was so nasty to him. She at first would not answer but with therapist prompting said, 'Because he tries to kiss me when he's drunk and says horrible things'.

Jim then accused Mona of 'falling to pieces inside' and only appearing to hold herself together so neatly. Others comment that Jim, in his guarded, obsessional way, is the one holding himself together and when drunk it all begins to come out—like the time he bit Jean in another kissing attempt.

The sexuality theme in the games played together is referred to by one of the doctors and Mary angrily dismisses this since, 'you're not here at night to know what's going on'. Julie says she can laugh at Bob's sexual feelings and not take them seriously. Mona and Jim both look aggrieved and Jim says he is frightened of his anger in situations like this. I suggest that his sexual and his angry feelings are mixed up together and that if he 'played', more and became involved with people perhaps disastrous things may not occur after all. Bill said he did not like all this talk of sex—'It's just warmth that people want.' Jack and Keith 'can relate to that' for they feel a need to 'fill a gap' (more laughter) and drinking alcohol somehow does this for them when no sexual relationship is available. I suggest that problems arise when infantile sexuality (with its simple closeness and warmth) is replaced by adult sexuality (with its physical actuality) and when that infantile sexuality of warmth and closeness is not adequately replaced 'it leaves a gap'. Julie says, 'we're all very Freudian today'—but agrees that adult sex, and warmth from and to people, get all mixed up in her and she cannot separate them—and 'maybe that's why I can't bear to touch people'.

Jean says that even sharing a pot of tea with someone is seen as a sexual approach here and she is dismissive of the topic. Jim 'fears' the same thing. Others remark that on the outside, invitations to tea, the cinema or a drink, etc., are indeed openers to possible sexual contact.

I intervene again to say that we are trying to move away from the idea that a warm approach from one person to another is necessarily destined to end in adult sexuality.

Jean says that people are not direct in their messages—'it's confusing'.

The final announcement is that tonight there is an *Inter-Action group*—despite the 'reality testing' that this entails, and which everyone clearly understands, there are few takers.

Thus, a meeting that is originally apparently concerned with social control in the unit has implications much deeper in the area of infantile sexuality. Most people in the room were involved actively or at least as interested listeners. By throwing the discussion about, drawing in this person and relating to that incident, the topic is not particularly seen as threatening and it never lost its contact with the actuality of the living situation. It remains meaningful to the current life together. No dramatic 'cures' are achieved and the group has to be set in its context to appreciate what value it might have been. Thus, in the succeeding small groups some of the patients returned to the theme; on other days reference back to the theme was made, particularly by Julie, who talked of her confusion when confronted by the affectionate demands of her own children in which she feared 'something sexual'. Jack was confronted with his habit of drinking milk from the bottle—'like a baby', 'the mess' in the unit was alluded to, and Stan asked if 'you all want your mothers to clean up after you'. Dependency on the staff remained a feature for some time; it had to be pointed out, and greater self-responsibility fostered, with staff urged to hold back from supplying all the answers in dynamic interpretations.

Psychotherapy in the large group can be a *facilitative* process if many members are drawn in and 'here and now' incidents related to possible neurotically held drives and feelings. When the group turns on one individual, however, and showers him or her with interpretation, opinion and exhortation it becomes *obstructive* and is entered into by the group as a *fight/flight* mechanism to escape from their own and other considerations. The staff must be particularly aware of this and hold the balance between sociotherapy and psychotherapy (Whiteley, 1974). Too much emphasis on psychotherapeutic interventions gradually leads into a situation in which the other staff feel even less capable of competing with the doctor psychotherapist—who might well then respond in the *prima donna* way with even more analytic interpretations. Then, the patients simply wait dependently for the next wise statement and group progress is halted. The patients assume a passive role waiting to be cured. The psychotherapy has become *obstructive*.

Contrived groups: the large group in training

The training potential of the large group can now be mentioned further. Springmann (1974) has commented that the large group, open to visitors, allows contacts to be made between patients and outsiders and views to be exchanged which decrease the amount of rejection that the outside community might hold for the patients. The large group often presents an *in vivo* working model of psychological and sociological mechanisms in a way that the more structured and formalised small group cannot do. The experience of being in a large group of 'non-patient' peers induces the same regressive, competitive, exciting, crazy, infantile or panicky nihilistic feelings that patients frequently express in psychotherapy, almost as if one has been given an abreactive injection. The large group can provoke a simulated neurosis or even psychosis which gives mental health workers invaluable insight into symptom formation, e.g. the feeling of non-existence or, at best, devaluation, when no one responds to a remark made. Staff will often comment in training seminars or sensitivity groups that they 'haven't anything of importance to say in the large group', or to the senior staff member that 'you always say it first, anyway', demonstrating the same self-denigration and projection of all their good parts into the idealised leaders that the patients display.

The same awkward silences occur, looking to the leader for instruction, and crazy things are said just to make personal space and register one's existence. There is a personal excitement to speaking and taking part and then sometimes receiving a flood of hostility and when the anxiety-laden session finishes everyone breaks into animated chat over inconsequential things with his neighbour!

Much of the Kreeger, de Maré and Institute of Group Analysis interest in large groups in fact arose out of conference situations and experiential study groups in the large group setting (Skynner, 1971; Bournique and Bournique, 1975) as Bion's theoretical expositions grew out of a study group and the therapeutic possibilities followed.

Natural groups: industry

Finally, some comment can be made on *naturally occurring* large groups, which can be seen particularly in industry and organisations with an administrative function. Some of the phenomena of the large groups were perhaps unwittingly utilised by the Victorian mill-owners who housed their workers around the mill, even building model villages such as Saltaire (the Salts of Yorkshire) or Port Sunlight (Lord Leverhulme). Thus, identification with 'the works' is engendered. Loyalty or subservience to the employer, as it may be variously seen, is similarly fostered today with cut-price factory products for the factory worker, sports and social clubs so that the worker's whole life comes to revolve about his job and the social and personal network emanating from it. However, Mumby (1974), who worked with large groups in industry, commented that in an industrial organisation the only mass meetings that occur arise when the union call men out and that it is astonishing that organisations have not developed these methods for their own purposes! The anonymity of the individual in a large organisation, the lack of meaningful contact and relationships and the feelings of unreality and valuelessness that occur in a large group can also be present in such an organisation. While Mumby feels that departmental large group meetings might expose inadequacies, illustrate hidden stresses and promote a corporate identity with improved task performance, he acknowledges that the corporate identity could challenge both management and union power.

Leadership is a key issue in the naturally occurring group. The members operate for the most part in a limbo of unsure relationships and unclear purpose, waiting to be taken over by anyone who clearly and forcefully points the way whether for good or bad purposes. When the leader gives direction, however, he gives order and a model for action to the group members who, in the process of time, organise to destroy, replace or shrug him aside, before descending again into the leaderless mass waiting the next crusade and mobilisation for action.

Natural groups: organisations

Problem-solving in naturally occurring large groups has been described by Whyte (1967). He writes of the *labour relations model* where management and workers, although pursuing the same 'goal' of improved productivity, see the situation from different standpoints and achieve a resolution of their differences by a bargaining process. In a *bureaucratic model* there is an imposed hierarchy from above with little or no bargaining opportunity, and this is the model of the civil service, health service and indeed most hospitals. In the *community democracy model*, which is a popular one for social clubs, trade unions and district associations, a consensus or vote system is utilised to resolve differences and reach decisions. Whyte points out, however, that the membership of these latter organisations is often so apathetic that attendance and participation is poor and they can seldom function as ideologically intended. He makes the allusion that the community democracy model of a therapeutic community could be an inappropriate one for the actuality of that situation, which he likens to the industrial situation. Staff and patients are in pursuit of the same goal—but see it from different standpoints and therefore have different ideas as to how it is to be attained. He suggests that a labour relations model for bargaining between staff and patients would be a more appropriate conflict-solving mechanism in a therapeutic community and that the community democracy model in a hospital can be false and can actually cover up a hierarchichal bureaucratic model.

In the same article he alludes to the selection of the appropriate model for achieving change in large organisations or developing potential. Very commonly—indeed, as in the 1974 reorganisation of the National Health Service—a bureaucratic model is imposed from above with delegation downwards through subordinates, committees and supervised underlings until the bottom level—where the field work is carried out—is reached. By now, lines of communication are so stretched and intermediaries so many, that delays occur, information is blocked or peters out and feelings of isolation and worthlessness arise, particularly at the grass roots. A more appropriate model for such a reorganisation is to start at the grass roots by ascertaining what facilities, resources, actual needs and particular skills exist in any one district (or hospital or factory) and then linking these with liaison officers, only as necessary, to maximise their cohesive functioning and mutual interdependency. This liaisive level reports directly to top management, without the hierarchical tree of multiple branches that are so often unnecessary.

Experiential groups 7

The human potential movement

Under the title of *encounter groups*, a variety of techniques, some sound and others questionable, have come to be used since the mid-1960s, to 'expand human potential' and promote personal growth through new experiences. The Encounter movement has given something to the more formalised group psychotherapy processes in terms of directing attention to physical presentation of the self, body movement, person-to-person contact and non-verbal interaction. It has elaborated methods of intensifying or expressing feelings, clarifying fantasy and translating feeling into action. Nevertheless, the plethora of games, exercises and techniques has to be sifted through with caution, for some are merely sensational rather than sensation-arousing, e.g. the nude encounter, and the proper place of encounter methods in the group therapy field is probably more in the field of 'group therapy for normals' than in the treatment of the mentally ill.

Origins and development

Like group psychotherapy, the roots of encounter groups can be traced back to the twin seeds of psychoanalysis in groups and the theory of group dynamics. The term 'encounter' was coined by Carl Rogers (1973) to describe the *basic encounter* between one person and another when each began to experience the other as a real person in closer and more direct contact than ordinary life allows and without the customary inhibitions and social conventions that prevent the expression of genuine feelings, both positive and negative. Rogers, a psychologist working from a background of individual psychotherapy and counselling, gradually moved into the intensive group experience as a means of developing interpersonal communication and relationships when he was asked to train counsellors for work with the returning GIs following World War II. He experimented with the group as an experiential teaching and learning situation, drawing on the already developing work of Lewin and his followers at the Massachussetts Institute of Technology.

A much earlier development, which was a more direct descendant of psychoanalysis, occurred when Wilhelm Reich, in the 1930s, began to expound his theories of bodily function, somatic tensions and the imbalance of the autonomic nervous system in neurosis and mental illness and attempted to draw this awareness into Freudian psychoanalysis. Much persecuted by the psychoanalytic establishment, and indeed by the US Government, Reich became mentally ill and died in a prison psychiatric hospital. However the awareness of body sensations in emotional disorders has been revived by exponents of the bioenergetics (Liss, 1974) school, which concentrates upon massage, tension release, touch, relaxation, body sculpting, etc.

Also with roots in orthodox psychoanalysis is the Gestalt psychotherapy of Perls (Perls *et al.*, 1973) but in this technique fantasy, dreams and hidden preoccupations are acted out and brought into the conscious through a more directive approach than psychoanalysis would favour.

Moreno in the 1930s had also moved away from psychoanalysis to examine symptoms and emotional problems in the actuality of their social context, thus taking a stance between group analysis and group dynamics. He developed psychodrama and from this evolved role-playing, which has a place also in the Gestalt school.

Meanwhile, Lewin's work at the Massachussetts Institute of Technology developed steadily into T- (or training) groups for non-patients wishing to study interpersonal behaviour. Interpersonal exercises were developed into inter-group exercises in conferences organised by the Tavistock Institute and the University of Leicester, and finally such exercises have been elaborated into mini-society experiments where cultural and social group tensions can be examined.

The regular format of weekly group meetings of a determined and usually brief period has gradually been eroded in most of these 'new' approaches, so that one-group meetings or workshops consisting of many and sometimes variously functioning groups will meet over a week or a weekend as a workshop. The term 'marathon group' is used to describe groups lasting over, say, two hours and usually for five or six hours, but sometimes into forty-eight hours or more.

A customary practice in an encounter group is for the leader to go through a variety of exercises, drawing on all or most of these different theoretical approaches as seems to fit the mood of the moment. Most of them have much in common, such as the banning of interpretation; the owning of opinions, statements and attitudes; in terms of 'I' feel or think thus, rather than using the impersonal 'one' or 'you'; the freedom to act as one wishes in terms of touch or movement; and the *relative* non-direction of the convenor who himself participates in the group.

We can now look in more detail at the different techniques and then review the research findings and general consensus of their value in treatment and training.

T-groups

T-groups (T = training) or *sensitivity groups* as they are sometimes called are a product of the group dynamics studies of Lewin and the National Training Laboratories which was formed in 1947 in Bethel, Maine. The T-group was primarily a process-centred study group, and in this respect Bion and the Tavistock Institute contributed to the origins. The object was to study behaviour in groups in terms of leadership, authority roles and dynamics with a view to improving functioning in a wide variety of industrial, educational or social organisations. Secondarily, the interpersonal dynamics and functioning of individual members came to be examined but, again, largely in the context of their functioning within the group and the organisation to which the group contributed. The third development into the exploration of the more personal and 'out-of-the-organisation' life of the individual members moves more into the sphere of action of what have now come to be called 'encounter groups'.

In the field of mental health, therefore, the T-group or sensitivity group is more likely to be a staff activity in which the professionals, engaged together in the common task, will meet to improve their work functioning, their inter-communication and their interpersonal relationships in the working group and will see from, and give to, their colleagues feed-back on personality, behaviour and attitudes.

The technique employed is usually verbal interaction and the group is often a leaderless one. However, the latent hierarchies in the staff group, for instance in a hospital or unit sensitivity group, often result in the actual staff leaders being pushed into a covert leadership role and much of the discussion takes place around the conflict with or loyalties to the staff leaders in a transferential way. For this reason, it can be advantageous to bring in an outside T-group leader to direct the group, but the disadvantage of this is that, being unconnected with the organisation, he may not always be fully aware of what is going on in the actual work situation and can only comment on the broad mechanisms that he picks up in the 'here and now' of the T-group. One of the anxieties of staff taking part in a T-group is that personal material may be disclosed to work colleagues, while another is that if they do not take part in the T-group they will be regarded by the staff leaders as unwilling or unable to participate fully in the group treatment programme with patients. Ground rules for the T-group could then be made so that matters relating to the personal life (rather than the working life) of the member should be excluded and that participation is voluntary. One overwhelming factor, however, in favour of staff who work in groups with patients taking part in a regular T-group is that they can come to know at first hand the anxieties of confrontation, the awkwardness of silence, the perplexity of not being answered, or the embarrassment of being excluded. In other words, they can experience and learn what it is like to be in a group.

The outcome of T-groups in terms of enhancing organisational efficiency, however, is summarised by Campbell and Dunnette (1968) from a review of the literature as 'neither confirmed nor disconfirmed'. In terms of translating what the members might have learned in the group into the 'back home' situation, the same authors conclude that 30–40 per cent exhibit some sort of perceptible change.

Group relations exercises

In 1957 a conference jointly sponsored by the University of Leicester and the Tavistock Institute set up a pattern for succeeding group relations exercises in this country and the United States. The original Leicester conference was described by Trist and Sofer (1959) as aimed at encouraging in those who participated a constructively analytical and critical approach to the way they performed their roles in the groups to which they belonged. The exercises followed on Bion's work and were a part of the developing group dynamics school. From 1962 to 1968 A. R. Rice of the Tavistock Institute headed the annual conferences and more clearly defined the purpose. In order to understand man in society it is necessary to shift one's view from the individual and the pair to the larger whole and take in the total perspective of the individual in his relationship to the many groups and sub-groups with which he is connected as if in a moving panorama. Rice (1965) directed attention first at understanding leadership and later at understanding authority. Rice described the primary task of the group as the function that it must carry out in order to survive. The study then becomes one of how the members relate and interact in the achievement of the primary task. As the Leicester conferences developed, so did interest widen from the study of the small group to the study of the total conference, the relationship of the sub-groups, and indeed of the conference, to the outside society. It became a global study of the influences impinging on the individual. While the Leicester conference studied leadership and authority, it is possible to designate another study topic as the primary task and focus upon that.

The conferences are residential, and last for about fourteen days, consisting of between fifty and seventy members. There is thus an optimal situation for the membership to concentrate upon the 'here and now' of immediate experience. One of the major aims is to contribute to people's ability to form serious work groups committed to the performance of clearly defined tasks. The sessions each last an hour and a half and are attended by a staff consultant. There are *four major exercises:*

(1) small groups of between eight and twelve to study their own behaviour;
(2) large groups of all the staff and student membership;
(3) inter-group exercises to study the relationship between groups, who operates for whom, and how delegation and representation comes about, etc.;
(4) application groups, in which those who actually work together or in allied fields study how they may apply the lessons learned in the 'back home' situation.

While the students are free to make of the meetings what they will, the staff maintain firm rules of punctuality and leadership directing attention to the primary task and making the members aware of what is going on in the group. The purpose is educational and not therapeutic and a trend to 'psychotherapeutic' disclosures would be explained as hindering the execution of the primary task. Thus the whole exercise bears relationship to Bion's study of the basic assumption groups. The emphasis is on the group not the individual, and therein is a major difference from the T-group. Learning and work, rather than personal growth or self-expression, is the aim that thereby differs from encounter groups.

Latterly, the Leicester conference style has been utilised with business delegates, academics, politicians, and the leaders of social and racial sub-groups (Rioch, 1970).

The mini-society

A development from the Tavistock Institute's study of the inter-group processes has been the study of inter-group tensions and sub-group formation in society at large. These exercises have been carried out in England and in Denmark by Gurth Higgins (1972), Hjeholt and others. Essentially, a volunteer community is brought together for a day or a few weeks and provided with the basic resources for survival, i.e. food and shelter. The overall community, however, is divided at the outset into sub-groupings which reflect a real division in social status. Thus, they may be the old and the young, male and female, the wealthy and the poor, the teachers and the students or various combinations of these naturally occurring differentials. The groups are given a task of studying their interaction and staff leaders are assigned as in the Leicester conferences. For each group problems of organising their own space in the exercise ground, designating themselves by a title and then negotiating with the other groups for the available material resources and arranging the conjoint study programme quickly emerge. Rivalry, competition, hostility, alliances, submission or rebellion become issues that have their parallels in the outside society.

There are no particular rules or programme of activities save for the following.

(1) A strict boundary of reality is drawn between the mini-society and the outside society. Within the bounds the members may do as they wish but their activity cannot spread over the

boundary line. A staff member keeps this boundary, both physical and metaphorical, in the minds of the members.

(2) The participants must agree to research their behaviour which is the object of the exercise.

Procedures for the opening stages may be suggested by staff, e.g. (1) the meeting of the sub-groups; (2) negotiating the boundaries in inter-group meetings; (3) meetings of the total community and (4) a pure research and review session; but once started, the participants make their own plans.

One common finding is that sub-groups tend to caricature their own roles in society initially, but then may attempt to escape the labelled role and negotiate for a different form of recognition. Other reactions are to rebel totally and be left with no identity, or to re-entrench within the accustomed role.

In a mini-society exercise at Henderson, probation officers were separated into (1) the younger male graduate entrants; (2) the older and more established male officers; and (3) the women probation officers.

The group dispersed to find names and territory and the women reported back first to say that they were 'Group No. 1' and based in the large meeting room! An hour or so later when the three groups convened the women were found to have moved to a smaller room, changed their name to 'the waiting-room group' and were making tea for everyone. Their experience had been that, when they sent a messenger to report to the older officers as they had done to the staff, the former had replied, 'No, no—*we* are the No. 1 group and shall be meeting in the large room', at which the women backed down. As the exercise continued the women found no alternative to their accustomed secondary and providing role; the older officers stuck rigidly to accustomed ground, while the young graduates, who called themselves 'the babies' and met in the attic room, played out a teasingly rebellious game with the old hands but at the same time did attempt to introduce and use innovative techniques throughout the week-long exercise.

The basic encounter of Rogers

The *Rogerian basic encounter* (Rogers, 1973) arose out of the Lewin T-group methods, influenced by the Gestalt psychology approach to the 'whole' person rather than his parts (or symptoms) and owing much to the style of so-called *client-centred psychotherapy* that Rogers (1957) had already developed.

In client-centred therapy Rogers seeks to convey 'unconditional positive regard' to the patient (client), empathise with the patient and communicate to him this genuine understanding and an acceptance of him without conditions.

In the basic encounter group the leader is designated a *facilitator*. He takes part in the group, openly expressing his own problems and difficulties as they may come to the surface. His role is to generate a psychological climate of safety in which mutual trust can arise and positive and negative feelings will be expressed. He makes clear at the outset that the group is free to make of the session what it wishes. The relaxed informality of the session may be further induced by simply sitting casually around the room on floor cushions or actually moving and milling about the room as the opening conversation moves and mills through the awkward introductory phases. The facilitator should listen attentively to whoever is speaking and at the same time try to empathise with the feeling component of the message. He will accept whatever it is that the individual or the group wishes to do or say without criticism but will influence the group to concentrate on 'here and now' experience and feelings, reactions to each other and feed-back to and from the other members, and will give feed-back to members of his own reactions to them. Interpretive or group process comments are avoided since they tend to depersonalise the individuals making up the group and distance the interpretation-giver from the others. Members are encouraged to say how they feel and think in the first person singular—e.g. '*I* feel. . . .' Physical movement and contact is not taboo, so that someone crying may be taken into the comforting arms of another person—even the arms of the group leader. While exercises or structured games are not imposed on the group to create effect, where appropriate such a physical situation may be constructed. A group unable to get together and break through their politely defensive interchanges may be open to a suggestion that they link arms and speak face-to-face to their neighbour, or it may be put to a group unable to trust each other that they form a circle and gently toss a colleague around the group in a way that he has to put trust in them that they will not 'let him down'. Role-playing situations arise fairly spontaneously in terms of one member saying to another, for example, 'you remind me of my father . . .' whereupon the facilitator may say, 'let him be your father—say what you want to your father—and listen to his answers back'. The phases that an encounter session or series of sessions goes through is much the same as in group analysis. The getting-to-know-people phase is followed by some resistance to participation and then often by the expression of negative feelings. Past memories are recalled, and the more immediate feelings and events are concentrated upon. Trust and mutual support develops and defensive facades are dropped. Feed back and confrontation can take place and change can result as comments are accepted, and more positive feelings can now find expression without anxiety.

Rogers warns against the facilitator who pushes the group towards goals *he* sets rather than the ones they do, or who seems to aim primarily for dramatic happenings. The facilitator who wants to be the centre of the stage, either with his problems or because he wants to organise the group into specific exercises, or who can pursue only one line of approach, is equally condemned as is the facilitator who withholds himself entirely aloof as the expert commentator rather than as a personally participating member.

Despite the protestations to the contrary, however, there can be little doubt that the personality and charisma of the encounter group leader is an important factor in getting the group to work, often very quickly, through a number of anxiety-laden emotional situations. The atmosphere of psychological safety is created largely by depending on the leader who is much more directive than, for instance, the 'conductor' in group analysis, and if the session continues for two or three hours or is part of a several-session workshop over two or three days, which tends to be the encounter pattern, the leader is invested with a great deal of awe and positive feeling.

Bio-energetics

Body language is commonplace. Words will 'stick in the throat' or excuses 'can't be swallowed'. Some incidents make us feel 'sick in the stomach', people give us 'a pain in the neck' or even 'take the piss' out of us. Body posture was remarked upon by Reich (1949), who wrote that 'the how of saying things is as important material for interpretation as is what the patient says', referring to the facial expressions, gestures and gazes. Defensive people will sit locked up in the group with arms folded and legs crossed. Remarks may be made through a constantly smiling visage in one who is fearful of rebuke whatever the content of the message. Reich introduced body therapy into psychoanalytic treatment by getting patients to yell out, pressing on their chests to release the 'knob of anxiety'. He also commented on the sympathetic and para-sympathetic imbalance in the autonomic nervous system, which is a contributory factor in the aetiology of the so-called stress disorders such as asthma, peptic ulceration, colitis and eczema.

The sympathetic nervous system was identified with the unpleasant anxiety and fear functions and the para-sympathetic with the pleasure functions—sexuality and the allayment of anxiety. The balance of the two autonomic functions, their relationship to sensory input via cutaneous and muscle receptors and their effect on muscle tension, vascular tone and heart rate is of more importance.

Bio-energetics is the name of the science developed by Lowen (1966) out of Reich's work to reach emotional states and achieve psychotherapy via body exercises. Such exercises will usually take place in the group with the assistance of all present, either as a body therapy session in itself or as part of a longer-running encounter group when, for instance, defensive awkwardness prevails at the beginning of the group or a particular patient seems to be 'holding back' on his aggression or, at the end of a group, when wind-down relaxation is called for. The group may be invited to become aware of their bodies by stretching exercises, standing their ground, or expanding their chests to shout.

They may imitate another person's posture to get into how he is feeling or pound a pillow to let out inhibited feelings of aggression that they might feel for some real-life individual. What does another member's posture tell us ? Has he got all the troubles of the world on his back, his nose to the grindstone or head in the clouds ? Do it and feel it. Janov (1970) elaborated on the expression of pent-up feeling through the voice, getting patients to talk directly to the important figure in their lives as if they were present rather than just relating the incident to the other members. To enhance the need to express feeling Janov would isolate the patient for twenty-four hours before the session and push for maximal emotional expression through direct talk, child talk, baby talk and 'the primal scream', the first emotive and primitive expressions between child and parent when words failed or perhaps were not yet formed, but the feeling was and is there still. In this acting through the early infantile experiences Janov is running parallel to the more orthodox psychotherapists who seek verbal reconstruction of the early emotional life, but Janov dogmatically refrains from the latter.

Touch and massage in the group are again aimed at communicating basic messages, such as 'comfort me' or 'hold me secure', or resolving the knotted musculature of tensed-up individuals. We sexualise touch and skin contact with growing adulthood, whereas in infancy the warmth and softness of the body is a comforting and pleasurable sensation without overtones of guilt and anxiety. *Soft-touch therapy*, developed by Boyesen (1970), involves gentle, circular, rhythmic massage movements with pauses between, in which the patient may free-associate as relaxation proceeds. Rolf has developed a deeper massage therapy (rolfing) in which each part of the body is massaged hard with fingers and knuckles and, again, memories and association are encouraged to be brought up. *Rolfing* (Schutz, 1971) is intended to re-integrate the body parts, stretch and release cramped-up muscles and realign the spinal column, opening up a pelvis closed off from the world or, in another way, to get at the emotional problems that have finally brought the individual to a cramped-up and tense posture; by working on the end results to the body, it is hoped to get to and remedy the basic disorder.

Gestalt therapy

Gestalt therapy derives its name from Gestalt psychology, which perceived objects or situations for their 'wholeness'. A visual stimulus is made up of the figure and the background and may be perceived differently according to which aspect of the total picture is concentrated upon. Fritz Perls, a psychoanalyst with a Freudian training, founded his theory of Gestalt therapy on the insistence of the need to consider the organism in relation to its environment as a 'whole' (Perls *et al.*, 1973). Thus, the breather cannot be studied without awareness of the air he breathes. Body and mind must be studied in the whole person, and the Gestalt therapists pay particular attention to the body as did Reich. When exploring an idea or a perception the Gestalt therapist asks the patient to study the minutiæ of the perception and to look at it from all angles in order to build up a composite picture. Attention is given to what is 'here and now', rather than to what is past or what may be in the future. If a proposition is made, the subject is asked to consider also the opposite and thus explore how he came to opt for one action and not its opposite. He is asked to bring into his awareness the conflict between *impulse* and *resistance*, which is an inner and unconscious conflict. The patient is made a student and an experimenter in his own investigation of the self. Body tension is considered to be due to the unaware manipulation of muscles in response to mental conflicts, and awareness gives relief, according to Perls.

Although deriving much from Freudian theory, Perls is critical of some psychoanalytic tenets and procedures. Thus, he sees free association as wandering away from the 'here and now'. Resistances, which in a Freudian analysis would be broken through, Perls sees as a creative product of the mind which should be understood and incorporated into the wholeness of the individual's psyche. Indeed, in this aspect he is leaning somewhat towards the Jungian point of view of a creative rather than a reductive analysis.

Although the practice of Gestalt therapy is not confined to groups, Perls and his associates had a considerable influence on the growing encounter movement at Esalen, moving that towards the 'here and now' experience and rather away from the more traditional T-group type of exploration and exercise. Thus, Gestalt exercises or techniques to increase awareness, perceive the opposites, and consider the fragments that go to make up the whole have been incorporated into encounter group sessions. On the whole, however, the Gestalt-ist works individually with a patient, although in the setting of a group, and other patients may be drawn in to comment, assist, relate or identify and in their turn participate in a therapeutic dyad with the therapist. For this, the group will sometimes encircle two central chairs in one of which, 'the hot seat', sits the patient who wants to work on a problem, facing the therapist. The latter draws attention to posture, grimaces, the *how* of expression, the messages that the body is giving to the mind and vice-versa. The parts of the body may be asked to talk to the mind.

'My back is killing me', says the patient.
'What does it say ?'
'I'm hurting because I have to sit you up straight.'
'Why do you have to do that ?'
'Because I have to keep you together. If I don't keep tight control the body will collapse and break up.'

In relating an incident or a memory the patient will be asked to recall the exact details—what did he take in; what went to make up the scene that somehow was registered as so hurtful?

Dreams are analysed in much detail with the patient being asked to role-play the parts of the dream. If the roof falls in he may be asked to speak out the part of the patient in the bed (ill, fragile) then of the bed (enclosing, faithful, warm) and then of the roof (hard, threatening, not holding up too well).

When decisions were made or action taken the conflict is brought to the awareness by asking the patient to let his 'top dog', the self-righteous, pushing and controlling part of his personality, argue it out with his 'underdog', the weaker, uncertain, questioning part of himself. As he does this he may switch from chair to chair composing a dialogue with himself.

Perls looks for the 'unfinished business' of previous experience, i.e., the uncertainties, anxieties, confusion and doubts left by experiences that were not in themselves whole, completed and satisfactory and thus assimilated into the personality as stable contributory parts. The 'unfinished business' is the seed of later neurotic symptoms which intrude into the 'here and now' experience and which have to be detected, explored and worked through to a satisfactory conclusion.

Psychodrama and role-playing

Psychodrama was developed by Moreno (1946) in the 1930s out of his dissatisfaction with traditional psychoanalysis and his opinion that placing the patient in the actuality of his social context was of major importance. He introduced methods of *sociometry*, measuring how other people in the group saw the individual, and encouraged people to react spontaneously to their fellow patients without the cloaks and disguises of inhibition and social convention.

Psychodrama can be introduced into treatment in many ways. During the course of a group it may be suggested that an individual role-plays the situation he is trying to recall. Others will take on the roles of the real people involved and the feed-back they give him may open up avenues for further reflection on his own behaviour. Or someone else can mirror the patient's behaviour and let him know how he looks or sounds. Let him be his father and have to deal with a kid like himself. After the real-life enactment one may suggest that he tries it another way and see what response he then gets from the bystanders.

More formally, a session may be set aside for psychodrama in which a script, usually taken from the life-story of one of the group, is roughly worked out. The individual who is to feature picks out his co-actors and broadly tells them what attitude this or that person would take. The essence of the session, according to Corsini (1966), however, should be on *spontaneity*, quick 'free-association' responses, so that emotional expression is released; *simultaneity*, so that many people are involved in a lot of interactive reactions to the main events at the same time and the wholeness of the situation impinges on the actor; *veridicality*, whereby the situation becomes so true to life that real-life reactions take over and the individuals are no longer playing out Bill's row with his wife but are rowing with Bill.

After such a session, some form of wind-down discussion is necessary to try to place in context the emotional issues that have emerged and to suggest alternative and corrective attitudes. Value may result from the pure abreaction, but social learning involves some conceptualisation of what has gone on between those involved.

A more structured form of role-playing may take place in training for social skills, when patients in the group, and before the critical appraisal of their fellows, go through the motions of applying for a job, dating a girl or even making a telephone call.

Role-playing interventions are of value in large groups and therapeutic community meetings where, indeed, patients are playing through roles, e.g. as chairman of a meeting or ward representative. A particularly punitive chairman may be getting a hostile silence from the group until one suggests to him that another type of approach could elicit a more co-operative response and 'why not try it out?'

Co-counselling

Re-evaluation counselling—later to be abbreviated to *co-counselling* (co = co-operative)—was originated by Harvey Jackins (1965) in Seattle in 1950. As a group therapy it is only a transient experience, since the actual process is conducted between two people, but it is common for a co-counselling trainer to get together a group of ten to twelve people initially and, in one or two instruction sessions, teach them the rudiments of the technique which they then go off in pairs to carry out. One individual may select another from the group as his partner for a number of sessions at weekly intervals, but it is also permissible to him to arrange to see another member of the group in concurrent sessions. The original group may re-meet at intervals to renew contact. Co-counselling sessions, however, may also take place during the course of an encounter workshop, which lasts several days and utilises a variety of techniques.

Summarised briefly, co-counselling consists of emotional release through verbalising the tension-arousing problems or incidents. There is no discussion, advice-giving, interpretation, censure or exchange of opinion. The role of the listener in the session is to give 'free attention' and thus facilitate the outpouring of emotion. A session lasts for two hours. In the first hour the talker talks and the listener listens and at the end of the hour they reverse places. It is a peer situation without the induced or expectant dependency of the usual psychotherapeutic procedures with a professional. In order to maximise the expression of feelings the listener must give his full attention to both the content and manner of the talk and rely on a few simple cues and prompts to keep the talk in a relevant and productive stream of thought. He is asking the talker to re-examine the dilemma or problem that he is conceptualising. The listener will stay largely silent but facing and looking at the talker with eye contact. When talk dries up he may give a 'come on' sign with his hand, nod expectantly, repeat or half-repeat the last statement made. If he detects a key phrase that the talker seems to have difficulty in getting out he may suggest that the talker repeats and repeats that phrase e.g. 'I could have hit him', until it gets easier to say. If the talker appears hesitant to say something—or seems to seek permission—the listener will encourage him. If he becomes bogged down in 'bad' feelings the listener may suggest that he revert to an earlier and easier stage of the session when he was talking about 'good' things until he can give freer expression to the 'bad' bits. When the voice drops to say shameful things the listener asks him to shout it out loud—repeating. Self-depreciation may result in the listener asking him to contradict these self-depreciating statements. 'I'm self-centred'—'I'm *not* self-centred'. The self-appreciation aspects of the session are important in helping the talker to revalue himself. Memory-scanning is a way for the listener to get the talker to go over the incidents and trivia of the day that finally added up to the depression or tension of which he complains—'Talk about yesterday—all day—you get up at 8—and then. . . .' he may say. Observing the talker's face and posture gives the listener clues as to the emotion-laden topics. He may notice a clenched fist and suggest the talker concentrate on his fist, what it wants to do—to go through these motions—or to do the opposite and relax the fist and put on a different expression. The session is abreactive and simply facilitated by the listener. The talker works on his own problem with the support of his co-counseller.

The key issues for the listener are (Liss, 1974b):

(1)   don't interrupt the flow;
(2)   keep the talker speaking for himself (*I* felt rather than you feel);
(3)   keep the conversation direct (if he is talking *about* his wife ask him to talk as if *to* his wife);
(4)   change rhetorical questions to statements of present feeling (Why did she do it ?—I feel put down by her);
(5)   change the complaining statements about others to *I* messages about how it makes the talker feel;
(6)   change negatives to definitives (I'm not feeling good—I feel lousy);
(7)   intensify expression by getting the talker to repeat or shout out key statements, carry out the physical act or exaggerate the facial expression that goes with the mood.

Transactional analysis

Transactional analysis (TA) was originated by Eric Berne as a method of psychotherapy applicable to both individual and group situations. Briefly summarised, TA depends upon the subdivision of the personality into *parent*, *adult* and *child* parts which are the attitudes and behaviourial patterns assimilated by the individual from different stages in his life. Thus, the parent aspect is the collection of attitudes and impressions taken in from the influence of the parents in the first five years of life. The child aspect is that simultaneously experienced and recorded in the mind emotional reaction to the various early life situations. From about ten months or so, the individual commences the process of self-actualisation and independent being which ultimately results in him being able to take independent action. To some extent, the adult monitors and tests out the parent and child attitudes, and when aspects are in conflict with each other one or other state will be said to be *contaminated* and thus not responding in a clear way. Very early in life the infant works out how he stands in relation to those around him and Berne describes four life positions (Harris, 1973):

(1) I'm not O.K.—you're O.K.—the dependent child.
(2) I'm not O.K.—you're not O.K.—the uncertain, insecure child.
(3) I'm O.K.—you're not O.K.—the child withdrawn from unstable parents.
(4) I'm O.K.—you're O.K.—the child in a stable parental relationship.

The attitudes taken up and the behaviour represented in the first three years of life then repeats in the interpersonal situations of later life—a *life script* is written.

In transactional analysis the life script, the positions taken up and the different aspects of the PAC (parent–adult–child) attitudes are analysed in a somewhat mechanistic way with the aim of giving the individual a further free choice of future behaviour. The freedom is gained through knowledge of how the parent and child attitudes are feeding into and influencing current behaviour. In interpersonal behaviour the parent, adult or child parts of an individual talk to the parent, adult or child parts of another. When communications are parallel i.e. when P talks to P and P responds to P,

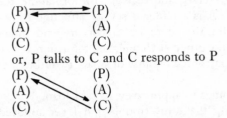

(P)⇌(P)
(A)   (A)
(C)   (C)

or, P talks to C and C responds to P

(P)   (P)
(A)   (A)
(C)   (C)

the communications are *complementary* and in harmony or collusion. When communications are crossed, i.e. when A talks to A but P responds to C, then

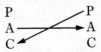

P   P
A————A
C   C

and useful communication ceases.

Transactional analysts regard the group situation as the most fruitful for treatment since the 'here and now' games being played out between the members can be analysed (Berne, 1966). The usual practice is for an individual to be instructed in the rudiments of TA theory and then invited to join the group for ten sessions, for instance. If he wishes to engage for a further period after that, this can be done but it is claimed that dramatic changes in life style can occur after only a few sessions. The goal for each member of the PAC group is clear, concise and easily stated, writes Harris (1973): to cure the patient by freeing his adult from the trouble-making influences and demands of his parent and child. The goal is achieved by teaching each member of the group how to recognise identify and describe the parent, adult and child as each appears in transactions in the group. The group leader, indeed, assumes something of a teacher role, sitting in one corner of the room and utilising a blackboard from time to time to illustrate the transactions that he and others may detect. The permissive, free-associating style of traditional psychoanalysis is thus not invoked since, Harris would have it, that is a child-to-parent transaction whereas what we are seeking is to speak adult-to-adult.

Berne (1966) regards a psychoanalytic training and a grounding in group dynamics as a preliminary to training as a transactional analyst and, although he avers that his subdivision of personality is different from the Freudian one of super-ego, ego and id, because the latter are concepts and the former is based on the physiological phenomena of actually perceived and registered information, the similarities are obvious. TA is a safe and sound, although somewhat mechanistic, way for the therapist to comprehend interpersonal reactions. In a large group at Henderson, for instance, one patient, Phil, was being confronted because of an angry outburst at the staff.

'I think you do these things to appear clever,' said Joan.

'I am clever,' said Phil, 'that's my trouble and I get annoyed when I see staff here getting paid who are not as clever as me and I can't get a job on the outside. The staff asked me how many staff members should come to the group—2 or 5—*adult to adult*—and then, when I gave a straight answer, they turned it all round and said I was over-dependent if I said 5 or trying to be independent if I said 2 and completely invalidated my answer.'

As a staff therapist I started to respond to his statement but other patients kept butting in, confirming that Phil's position was hopeless.

'You'll have to get a job as a comedian,' said Mandy.

At last I get a chance to speak.

'It sounds crazy if you have to come into a lunatic asylum [my exaggeration] to be clever whilst on the outside you held your job as a barman because you used to act mad [he was actually kept on in the bar as something of a freak]. Maybe there is a job—as hostel warden, group counseller or similar—where you could be clever and accepted as clever.'

To do this however, he will have to abandon his own C-to-P provocation, for one of the added reasons he got angry at the staff was because when he asked if he should take on the job as chairman of the community the staff member replied 'What do you think?' and didn't give a parental Yes or No answer.

In his book, Berne gives a series of comparative examples of statements analysed according to the different group theories. Thus, the question 'what are we supposed to do in the group?' would be answered encouragingly in a supportive group but dependency would probably ensue. A Bion-type interpretation might suggest a flight from taking the initiative. Ezriel would understand a move to the 'required relationship' of compliance with the therapist. Foulkes would see the individual surrendering his independence to the group's authority. Psychoanalysts might see in the question passivity and dependence, with the infantile sexual associations of this state transferred on to the analyst and the consequences defended against. The transactional analyst would understand the question as an opener to *the game of 'psychiatry'*. The patients would play along in the group producing the symptoms that the therapist would like to hear but on the outside continuing to preserve their own patterns of behaviour. His response therefore, would be to ask the patient why he poses this question and what he thinks he is supposed to do. Thereafter he will expound the contract and the theory of the TA group.

The Synanon game

In 1958 an ex-alcoholic called Chuck Dederich set up a 'free association' group with other alcoholics and addicts. It developed into an aggressively confrontative type of meeting and, as the community of addicts settled down together to live in first a house and then a hotel and finally a small community of houses with a self-supporting industry in California, Synanon was born. As this particular, peer-group-orientated way of life developed, so other non-addicts came to join or to visit and take part in the unique aspect of life at Synanon which is the *Synanon Game*.

The Synanon Community is divided into 'tribes' of between fifty and sixty people and the tribe is re-divided into sub-groups of twelve to sixteen members. Two to three times in the week, the sub-groups assemble for a 'game'. The room in which they meet is rather featureless so that it does not have the atmosphere or associations of a room used for social or business purposes, for instance. The members sit around the walls, often with a table intervening, and take part in a two-to-four-hour session of direct and aggressive confrontation on the 'here and now' observations of each other's behaviour.

The game is a verbal abreaction, an outpouring of intense emotional expression directed at one member of the group by the others in the blunt direct language that comes bursting to the surface. It is therefore, a repetitive, unintellectual, exaggerated and something of a sledgehammer technique but it must remain at a verbal level, and this is the contract that the game-players enter into. In the outpouring of spontaneously occurring expletives or impressions there is an in-built search for the fundamental aspect of one individual's personality or attitude and how this comes across to and affects other people.

Thus, a game in which a member is accused of slacking may simply go on,

> 'You're a bum!'
> 'I do as much as you!'
> 'A lazy bum!'
> 'A god-damned bum!'
> 'Bum, Bum, Bum . . . !' (screaming)

The Synanon Game was developed for the treatment of heroin addicts and its harsh confrontative nature, with narrow perspective and uncompromising limits, is appropriate in the management of the alienated, lost, empty personality of the addict, who needs tight management; but it has less to offer the general psychiatric patient to whom it could be damaging.

Encounter exercises

A large number of *encounter exercises* have now been described and Schutz (1973) recounts when and how they might be used in therapy. While some exercises are designed to focus on symptoms, e.g. muscle tension or a posture inadvertently held, others are aimed at tension release through abreaction. Conflict situations can be brought to light by going through some routinised exercises such as guided fantasy, or resolved through other experiences such as role-playing. Exercises should only be introduced for a purpose, however, and not simply as a time-filler. Some examples are as follows.

Body exercises, such as muscle tensing and relaxing, chest expanding by shouting, unlocking the folded arms and crossed legs, or *doubling*, in which other people portray in an exaggerated way how one individual holds himself, may draw attention to how the body as a whole is responding to and reflecting the mood.

Personal functioning is explored by fantasy dialogues between the two halves of an individual's mind as he tries to come to a decision. The individual speaks out loud the two sides of the conversation.

In a *guided fantasy* the group leader prompts the relaxed individual to elaborate on a fantasied topic e.g. 'you are standing on a narrow ledge—say what you feel—describe it—what's going on'.

Dream enactment similarly calls for the individual to recount a dream but taking in all the parts so that again we get some insight into his conflict of desires and fears.

Breaking in and *breaking out* consists of forming a tight circle of other group members and putting the individual outside or inside the group so that he experiences the feelings of alienation or constriction and has to respond to this by trying to get in or out of the circle. This is of use, for instance, for someone who feels an outsider or is unable to escape from a situation. After the exercise he might be asked to role-play a real-life situation which parallels the exercise.

Interpersonal functioning is explored through *milling*, when the group members wander about the room seeking someone with whom to relate. They might be asked to form dyads—and converse for two or three minutes about a good experience; to exchange non-verbal cues of reassurance; to take up positions that reflect how they feel about the others (or the leader) or to mill into groups for whom they feel affinities. *Blind-milling* is done with eyes closed, the members being asked to reassure or hug those they bump into and then pass on, so that a non-verbal message is conveyed.

Trust games are structured to induce the individual to relax and not hold back from people. Thus he may be taken on a blind-fold walk or be passed around the circle of outstretched hands while he passively accepts.

Sculpting the family or a recent situation with others, consists of one individual placing other people physically around the room as he sees the members of his family, for instance, in relation to himself. The situation can be intensified by the actors feeding-back how they feel at being thus positioned.

Group fantasy consists of the members lying down as in the spokes of a wheel and one after the other elaborating on a common fantasy.

After most or all of these exercises some period should be set aside for the members to describe how it felt. The leader may have to ask them directly or even to comment on what he observed. If a particularly bad experience was felt it might be suggested that they repeat the exercises but this time in a different way, being aware of and trying to overcome the particular difficulties that this member may have gone through.

Inter-Action games

Inter-Action Trust, founded by American-born actor and theatre director Ed Berman, provides a game-playing session of about two hours for a group. The numbers need to be between fifteen and twenty-five to create an atmosphere that can become animated and with which everyone can get involved. The group director must be unashamedly directive, dynamic and energetic in keeping the pace going and switching from one game to another as the mood seems appropriate or as expediency dictates. Sometimes it may be necessary to stimulate activity but at other times to ease down the tempo.

The session is essentially a game for enjoyment but one in which (as in all games) an element of fantasy, role-playing, experimentation or new experience can take place if the player wishes it. The game gives him permission to act out a part but the rules provide the controls so that fantasy and reality can be held in correct perspective.

The games are verbal and non-verbal, and designed to be points of contact between people, opening up *creative opportunities,* stimulating *competition* and encouraging *co-operation.* They have been used in situations where social contact is poor either for environmental or for psychological reasons. Thus, neighbourhood children may be drawn into contact through a street session, or withdrawn mental hospital patients may be stimulated to make contact.

Although a large number of brief games are included in the repertoire they depend basically upon

(1) *rhythm*—in sequence the members in a circle may clap, make a noise, or touch their neighbours. These games are usually used as ice-breakers;

(2) *tag*—through the physical contact of a touch the game moves from individual to individual, e.g. building up on an idea or a fantasy;

(3) *buck*—the principle is the same, in that an unwanted object is passed from one to another.

Examples of games used in the Inter-Action method are as follows.

Ice-breaking games are utilised to overcome the inhibiting social barriers between participants at the beginning of a session and would include such things as rhythmic clapping, making some sort of noise or gesture in sequence around the circle to express a point, collecting specified information e.g. names, place of birth, from the others, making one's neighbour laugh, imitating the expression of one's partner, etc. Following this, *concentration games* may be used to alert mental processes and induce participation and involvement. The members may have to shout out the name, place of birth, etc., of whichever member the leader points to. A shopping-list is added to by each member who must repeat the whole list in turn.

Personality games can be utilised with more sophisticated groups. A person leaves the room and others find three words to describe him. He must guess who provided these words. Members move towards those they like or dislike most on the ward concerned. Members imitate the mannerisms of another member. A member lines up the others in order of popularity, stability, sexiness etc. Members mill around the room and when instructed say one word to describe the person nearest to them.

Acting games involve more fantasy production. A member may be asked to do something, e.g. read a book in the manner of a selected adverb (e.g. 'clumsily'). In sequence the members add to a fantasy story by acting the next addition. A person is moulded into a posture which expresses how others see him. A puppet play is acted out with one person working the limbs of another while a third supplies the voice.

Eclectic encounter

The customary encounter group session now utilises a mixture of exercises drawing from bio-energetics, Gestalt, co-counselling, psychodrama and role-playing, interspersed with periods of more reflective discussion in the open and direct way of Roger's client-centred basic encounter groups. Such sessions are often one-meeting events lasting three to five hours and their value is debatable.

At Henderson we have settled for a pattern of encounter group that, likewise, draws on the various techniques already described but has certain ground rules appropriate to the situation. The encounter groups take place at weekly intervals and the members are drawn from an in-patient group of young adults with person-ality disorders who are already in large and small group therapy in the setting of a therapeutic community.

No one is allowed to join in the group until he has been in the unit for four weeks and has become a 'known quantity' to the other group members and, also, is someone who has committed himself to the treatment situation.

The group *is* selective, in contrast to Roger's non-selectivity, because we have found that the intensity of the group is such that particularly vulnerable personalities can become increasingly disturbed. Members are invited to join if they seem to need physical release, an opportunity for emotional expression, the dispersal of inhibiting or controlling impulses, or simply training in social skills and physical and verbal contacts with others. Encounter groupies who want to get in on yet another rediscovery trip would be encouraged to stay within the more reality-based therapy of the community.

The group consists of twelve to fifteen members, small enough for all to be involved continuously and in everything, yet large enough for anyone to be able to sink into the general group back-ground if he feels too prominent. The group is conducted by one staff member with two subordinate assistants. The conductor must be directive and forceful enough to carry the group with his authority and stability yet not be so dominant that it has no life of its own. For this reason, he is best chosen from the 'middle management' of the staff hierarchy, neither so lowly that he would be taken over by a patient sub-group, nor so high up that he would be invested with an awe and regard that stifled any free expression either from himself or from the other members.

The conductor must be able to take part in the group, as must his assistants, and in a group of patients also involved in more formal psychotherapeutic interchanges with the same leaders there are obvious problems. Transference and counter-transference issues will be present. Self-disclosure in this situation may lead to the expectation of such in another. Manipulative or frankly destructive acting-out can occur with the conductor/therapist in this new and assailable situation. The team of conductor and assistants can support each other in these situations and spread the emotional strain.

The session lasts a minimum of three hours and a maximum of five but the time is agreed at the outset so that events can be paced. The sessions run for four consecutive meetings in any one block and the participants are asked to contract to attend all the sessions. The meeting room is comfortable and warm and away from sight and sound of the rest of the community. Floor cushions take the place of chairs and the first session starts with a brief preamble about the aims, rules, timing, etc. The opening will then consist of body exercises to break out of stereotyped postures, expressions and attitudes. Stretching, shouting and general disinhibition can be achieved by an exercise such as 'Mad dog', where all in the group, as individuals but in concert, act out the situation where a mad dog has latched on to an ankle. Followed up by a 'Rolfing'-type back-pummelling in pairs, the group is now physically and mentally loosened up enough to move on.

They sit around and the conductor will ask what they want to make of the group, or what is preoccupying people. He may remark on what he observed of someone's participation in the exercise. He is looking for a lead into emotional exploration and unlike the group-analytic situation will try to short circuit a defensive silence. Although he and his assistants have access to a number of structured exercises he will not string the exercises one after another or introduce them simply to get things moving.

The exercises are utilised to amplify a point or stimulate alternative ways of behaving. A patient talking about his guardedness in the group may lead the conductor to suggest a *trust* exercise. The group forms a basket-like circle with linked arms in which the untrusting individual may be gently tossed from one to another. Others might like the experience and take a turn. Shyness and inability to make physical contact may be the signal for blind-milling, in which, with eyes closed, the members walk about the room and, if they bump into someone, indicate reassurance by hugging or squeezing and then move on. A brief co-counselling exchange may follow a complaint that 'no one listens to me'. Role-playing through a situation is always a frequent possibility, either in the very pointed Gestalt way of the hot-seat in the middle of the circle or simply and briefly during the course of a discussion. Involvement of other people and their spontaneous attitudes in the role-playing enriches the situation. Sculpting the family can be a way for someone to show what it's really like in his home. He positions people around the room in postures and places as they seem in relation to him, and then those so-positioned may be invited to give him a piece of their mind. For instance, a mother whom he has set up high on a pedestal but distanced from him, may protest that it is both unsafe and isolated up there and what she wants more than anything is to be down with the others. Talking and working through the session at a gentle pace, utilising the action to facilitate expression and not to provide a diversion, the group is both exploratory and cathartic, and material that comes to the fore or is seen in a different way through physically acting it out can be utilised further in the formal group-analytic sessions of ensuing days. The encounter session should not be seen as a specialised and self-contained entity in its own right.

The conclusion of the group should occupy the last thirty minutes and be a relaxing wind-down with decreasing verbalisation and recourse to comforting, supportive and group-cohesive exercises. Gentle massage, group hugs, milling with eyes open but with reassuring touches take precedence.

Evaluating encounter groups

The effect and impact of encounter groups has been controversially debated. Rogers (1973) claims that the intensive encounter group is 'perhaps the most significant social invention of this century'; but several US commentators and politicians warned against the 'brain-washing', 'sensitivity training for planned change' and other such dangers to the *status quo* that they feared from the encounter movement.

Rogers, quoting his own and Gibbs's (1970) follow-up studies of encounter participants, reports that the majority of participants felt the experience helpful, meaningful and having some lasting effect and that there was little basis for concern about the possible traumatic effects. Indeed, only 4 of 1,200 YMCA directors who had taken part reported a negative experience. Rogers is not selective or exclusive of subjects for the encounter group, discounting claims such as those of Gottschalk (1960) who asserted that they are 'psychiatrically disruptive to almost half the delegates'. Reddy (1970), however, partially supported the contention that sensitivity training could evoke pathological responses. Parloff (1970b), after reviewing the literature on encounter group results, states that whilst most participants report a positive response,

there is but little evidence that subjective changes are
enduring or that these changes are followed by behavioural,
personality, or performance improvements. As with any
intensive and emotionally stimulating experiences they result
in transitory emotional disturbances in some participants and
enduring pathological disturbances in a few.

Or more picturesquely, that 'participation in most encounter groups is likely to be more dangerous than attending an office Christmas Party and somewhat less dangerous than ski-ing'.

Cooper (1975), in similar vein and after a review of outcome studies, writes that there is no proven evidence that encounter groups are psychologically dangerous and they may be 'less stressful than University examinations or perceptual isolation experiments'. Hoerl (1974) comments somewhat ruefully, after an experimental examination of flexibility of attitudes in people attending encounter groups, that those volunteering for the sessions already had a high degree of flexibility and that this showed no great change as a result of the sessions. Many were already encounter groupers on a more or less regular basis and 'perhaps the people who could profit most from encounter groups are the individuals not attending them'.

On the positive side, though, it must be said that Parloff (1970b) views as one of the major contributions of encounter group practice for the analytic group therapist the development of procedures that facilitate rapid group formation and group cohesion. Cooper (1975) adds that the encounter group may enable participants to cope better with sexual and aggressive stimuli and stressful periods in their lives.

The incorporation of encounter techniques or the occasional intervention of an encounter group into ongoing group psychotherapy of a more formal nature is advocated by some writers, who see the encounter experience as providing an intensive affective experience (Parloff, 1970b) and a way of conceptualising immediate ideas which cannot be formulated in more conventional ways (Teicher *et al.*, 1974). Teicher, however, believes that encounter groups provide for what he calls *sociocultural deficiency states*, which is not the same as group psychotherapy which is aimed at *psychopathological states*, and adequate screening of both participants and group leaders is stressed and echoed by Reddy (1970).

The verdict of Lieberman, Yalom and Miles (1973) on encounter therapies is cautious and critical, however. After failing to initiate a field study of actual and current encounter groups they constructed a research exercise out of students attending a Race and Prejudice course at Stanford University. The 210 students were randomly assigned for thirty hours' participation to eighteen encounter groups of different modalities much as outlined in this chapter, and a control group of unassigned students was also followed; thus T-groups, Gestalt, transactional analysis, Synanon, psychodrama, Rogerian encounter, etc., were all represented as was a psychoanalytically orientated group. Assessments of outcome, both positive and negative, leader influence and group characteristics were made from self-report, reporting on each other, and questionnaires about social and personal interaction.

The findings can be summarised as follows:

(1) Sixty per cent reported immediate benefit but in a fifth of these it was not sustained. Self-evaluation tended to be higher than the evaluation given by others and by test results and the conclusion is that there was a 'modest positive gain'.

(2) A negative outcome in terms of persisting psychological disturbance was found in 7·5 per cent of those who began the course but some of these dropped out early. The casualties were not related to any one type of group, but leadership style seemed the crucial factor. Leadership styles could be categorised, whatever the ideological school—as aggressive, loving, *laissez-faire* etc.—and the casualties tended to result from the aggressively confronting, challenging, authoritarian but often charismatic figures who structured the group with high input of stimuli.

(3)   Learning resulted not just from the discharge of emotion but when this was associated with insightful thinking. Group exercises of themselves produced little of value.

(4)   A high output of anger was similarly not an essential for improvement; love and support were also needed.

(5)   While 'here and now' experience was valuable, so was recollection of the 'there and then'.

(6)   Groups that were cohesive, with agreed and established norms of behaviour, were more productive.

(7)   Any improvement that takes place shows up at once—there is no 'late blooming', but self-evaluation tends to be higher than actual results showed and gains tend to fade in an appreciable number.

(8)   Leadership is not such a change agent as is the influence of the group itself. Leaders who were neither aggressively directive nor passively *laissez-faire* did best. A moderate input rather than a high input of stimuli was best, and favoured techniques such as 'the hot seat' and other structured exercises have no relation to outcome. A leader who himself had some grasp of the group dynamics did best and his role was to create a climate that favoured both appreciation of 'here and now' experience and reflection on the past with some view of future functioning.

Strupp (1973), in an analysis of experiential groups which the authors of the 1973 review of group psychotherapy literature in the *International Journal of Group Psychotherapy* called 'one of the most important theoretical papers' (Reddy and Lansky, 1974), attributed the encounter movement's popularity to an essential value orientation which strongly contrasted with psychotherapy. Rather pessimistically, Strupp (1973) wrote that

> The traditional psychotherapeutic enterprise is on the decline because the moral and philosophical values implicit in its theoretical formulations are no longer in keeping with the prevailing view of man and his place in society. Conversely, the experiential group faithfully mirrors the aspirations, values, and needs of a growing number of people, and it seemingly offers solutions which the traditional therapeutic enterprise has failed to provide. Further, the process by which these solutions are achieved embodies a model of selfhood and interpersonal relationships seen as congenial or fulfilling by contemporary man.

8 The special application of group techniques: family therapy

The small psychotherapy groups so far described have been partially selected *stranger groups* in the main, where some effort was made to balance the group so that no one person was an isolate among others who had things in common. The idea of a 'balanced aquarium' of moderate differences in age, social class and symptomatology was sought after.

The fact that the members came to the group as strangers gave the initial exploratory processes some therapeutic purpose while the lack of prior knowledge allowed unbiased opinions to be formed.

However, there are instances when a more *selectively homogeneous group* may be formed in which the members have in common the principle ailment, e.g. as in a group of phobics, or the same general area of problem formation, e.g. as with adolescents, drug users, alcoholics or delinquents. In other respects the 'balanced aquarium' features still apply, but the group will clearly be occupied with finding mutual help in overcoming the shared problem.

A third form of specialist group is the *non-stranger* or *naturally occurring* group. In the field of group dynamics the T-group for members of a common work staff has already been described, but more important natural groups are the family or married couples which are discussed in the second half of this chapter.

Homogeneous groups

Group treatments of individuals with the same basic presenting symptom have been described in a variety of situations. The danger is that the group members simply relate to each other around the presenting symptom and discussion remains at a superficial level, largely confined to reminiscences of shared experiences.

Addicts exchange stories of the 'trips' they have made and alcoholics of their lost weekends. Such homogeneously selective groups may sometimes result from therapeutic desperation, the members being lumped together in an effort to find some common denominator which might provoke interaction of a therapeutic nature.

Alcoholics, addicts, delinquents and gamblers, particularly, have been referred to 'group therapy' although the positive evidence of the ability of these selected categories to utilise group psychotherapy to achieve insights and change is minimal.

Hand *et al.* (1974) reported on agoraphobics who were subjected to 'flooding', i.e. exposure to their travel or social anxiety precipitants. A group who were induced to develop some cohesion by discussing their mutual problem before the exposure, which was again carried out in a group situation so that the members could support and encourage each other, was found to be more successful in overcoming the problem than individuals who were not encouraged to discuss the problem initially and who were exposed to the phobia precipitant without the group support.

It is probably this same mutual support and encouragement, and peer group control, that alcoholics, addicts and gamblers particularly gain from each other, which is the crucial factor in accounting for the success of the organisational groups such as Alcoholics Anonymous and Gamblers Anonymous rather than any development of psychodynamic insights.

Addiction

For addicts there are community projects such as Synanon or Phoenix House, which have a strict code of discipline and techniques of harsh confrontation, which demand an almost ritualistic allegiance to a pattern of behaviour and which impose the controls from outside that the addict is unable to exert from within.

The Synanon Game has already been alluded to and the full Synanon living experience is described by Yablonsky (1967). In summary, it is a philosophy of living rather than a treatment process and has begun to attract other than addicts to its residential community in California where, once admitted, the individual may remain for life in a kibbutz-like organisation of self-help and mutual collaboration to the greater benefit of the somewhat unreal and isolated parent community. High motivation is demanded before an addict can be admitted and once admitted he renounces all drug contacts and indeed most of his external commitments as he becomes engaged in the 'tribal' activity of the community. A social system of positive living has been developed at Synanon in the belief that, if a particular social situation can produce a person's problems, another constellation of people operating within the framework of a constructive social system can ameliorate the same problem. Synanon remains an American institution with its parent settlement in Santa Monica, although there are now smaller subsidiary settlements in other centres.

The Phoenix House project for addicts had a somewhat different origin in that it was politically imposed by Mayor Lindsay of New York in 1968 as an alternative to the previous administration's detoxification programme for addicts (Small, 1974). Thus in three years it achieved the numbers that Synanon had grown to in ten years, but the strength of Synanon lay in its intrinsic culture and evolution whereas the Phoenix House philosophy was imposed from without.

In the UK a Phoenix House was established in London in 1970. The regime there is modified from the American experience but follows similar principles. A stated aim is the complete transformation of the former addict into a whole mature adult person and is outlined in the Information for Professionals (Phoenix House, 1971). A newcomer passes through an *induction* phase, in which he has to make contact with the centre himself, attend assessment meetings regularly, sever his contacts with other addicts and discontinue his intake of drugs. He is given encouragement by ex-addicts in the induction group but no material help. He has to make his own arrangements for attendance and thus his motivation is put to the test. *Residential rehabilitation* is commenced when he is off drugs and has thus proved his motivation. On admission he is given a lowly job in the hierarchy of the house, e.g. cleaning, and has to work his way up to management or administrative posts. A major factor in the treatment are the *encounters*, which are harsh, direct confrontations between the residents in which attitudes, differences and opinions are freely and forcefully expressed. They are both cathartic and insight-directed, much as in the Synanon Game. Acting-out behaviour is not allowed. The disturbed member is expected to take his grievance to the next encounter. Residents are also encouraged to 'act as if', i.e. to try themselves out in new roles in a positive way, rather than reiterating the negative aspects of their lives and personalities in the hope that eventually such behaviour becomes internalised. For example, a resident may be asked to 'act as if' he was responsible for keeping a newcomer off drugs and to put over the arguments and institute the check controls. The *re-entry* stage is the final stage before leaving, and now dependence on the group is lessened. The member is encouraged to make contact with people outside the house, possibly to assist in *induction encounters* or visit addicts in prison or hospitals to explain the method. Gradually he takes less part in the house activity and assumes studies or work training in preparation for life outside.

The Phoenix House programme is a mixture of behaviourist ('act as if') and insight (encounter) therapies (Small, 1974). A central feature is the attempt to transfer dependence on drugs to dependence on the house; this is assisted by the stress on an initial display of motivation, and once in the house it is reinforced by daily rituals in which the members chant together the House philosophy ('We are here because there is no refuge finally from ourselves . . .' etc. etc) and join in a cheer-leading type of acclamation ('What is the light of the world ?'—Phoenix!' etc.). Dependence to a degree of institutionalisation is aided by use of in-group language, terminology and catch-phrases for the various posts held (from 'crew' to 'ramrod' and thence to 'departmental head' and 'co-ordinator'). Breaches of the rules result in a snakes-and-ladders type of demotion even to the extent of being assigned to repetitive and degrading punishment tasks such as cleaning and re-cleaning the floor. Phoenix House is largely a peer group organisation staffed by ex-addicts who have 'made the grade', and the intention is that outside psychiatrists or other specialist consultants are only called in to advise as the members deem it necessary. A degree of dependence on the house remains for many who succeed to the final stage of becoming staff members despite the intent that members at the re-entry stage should gradually phase out, and the houses can be criticised (Small, 1974) for their tendency to induce conformity through discipline rather than personal growth through insight and theory. Small (1974) reports that, of the first 100 entrants, 71 left against advice, 8 were discharged for misdemeanours, 2 transferred to hospital and 1 was sentenced to prison; 13 completed re-entry, leaving 5 still in treatment at the time of the study. Of the re-entrants, 4 were employed in the House, 4 were in similar projects elsewhere and 1 was contemplating such.

Alcoholism

The group treatment of alcoholics stems from the pioneer work of *Alcoholics Anonymous*, which convenes large regional meetings with a supportive and educational purpose and smaller and more intimate ongoing district meetings which similarly provide support, encouragement and mutual self-help for the members, not only at the weekly meeting but also in between meeting times. Members have access to each other at any time and new members are given an older member as a guide and mentor to call upon in crisis. There is both a ritualistic and a religious basis to an AA meeting which supplies the element of external control that the alcoholic requires. He is expected to renounce alcohol absolutely and for life, but also to view his future in terms of getting through the next twenty-four hours without a drink. The 'twelve steps' downward from social drinking to helpless alcoholism are pointed out diagrammatically and in group exhortations, and the corresponding steps upward to sobriety are indicated.

The complex and multi-factorial aetiological factors in alcoholism are pointed out by Glatt (1974), who was largely instrumental in the UK for introducing group and milieu therapy programmes into the treatment of alcoholism. Glatt made an early alliance with AA groups and succeeded in involving alcoholics in hospital treatment in AA meetings outside the hospital to lend support to the specific treatment programme, whether the latter was physical treatment, aversion therapy or group psychotherapy. While most alcoholic treatment courses utilise a form of milieu therapy to render immediate support and some control over drinking, the effects of more intensive group and analytic psychotherapy are equivocal.

One paper reviewing various treatment approaches with alcoholics, including aversion therapy, group treatment and a simple ward regime, concludes that 'the outcome . . . depends very little upon the treatment given but largely upon individual factors relating to each patient and upon the natural history of the condition' (McCance and McCance, 1969). Very similar conclusions are reached by Rathod *et al.* (1966) after a two-year follow-up of males treated mainly with in-patient group therapy and compared with results from other treatments. 'One is almost tempted to suggest', they say, 'that, on the whole it is not so much the type of treatment which determines outcome but how efficiently it is carried out.'

Kissin *et al.* (1967) reported no difference between alcoholics treated by milieu therapy, group psychotherapy or drug therapy, although all improved significantly when compared with an untreated control group.

Most treatment procedures in the UK liaise with Alcoholics Anonymous, which can provide a supportive and encouraging network for many which then makes it possible for more specific or individualised treatments to be carried out and gives the individual the impetus to persevere with the treatment outlined. Parallel organisations for the wives and families of alcoholics correspondingly give support, encouragement and education about the problem and its treatment.

Delinquency

Although Arnold and Stiles (1972) reported a rapid increase in the use of group therapy in penal institutions, saying that it was one of the most widely used therapeutic techniques in such institutions, they also showed that many 'therapists' were largely untrained, groups were increasing in size for organisational reasons and were often essentially *repressive–inspirational* in character, i.e. controlling and counselling rather than insight-giving.

The group treatment of delinquents is largely based on residential therapeutic community experiences, and as such has already been referred to in chapter 4.

There is, of course, a long history of such 'living and learning' group techniques deriving from work with juvenile offenders and maladjusted youths. In the postwar years the Maxwell Jones (1962) methods were adapted to work in penal settings and particularly in the California Department of Corrections. Douglas Grant, working in a US naval detention centre at Camp Elliott, had studied both inmates and therapists engaged in group interactions. To summarise briefly, he divided his therapists into high (believing in a psychodynamic orientation) and low (relying on regulations and discipline) maturity subjects as he did his prisoner inmates. The findings after a period of group 'living and learning' experiences, in which therapists and inmates interacted in both activity and discussion groups over some weeks, was that high-maturity offenders responded well to high-maturity therapists, and low-maturity offenders responded well to low-maturity therapists, but low-maturity offenders did badly with high-maturity therapists and high-maturity offenders did badly with low-maturity therapists.

Building on these findings, Grant developed a scale of I-(integration) levels from 1 to 7 to guide future planners, and Jones suggested that the ideal offender-patient for a therapeutic community programme would be a short-sentence first offender, with a relatively high social maturity (I-level) rating.

In fact, a therapeutic community in a penal situation was set up at Chino, California, in 1958, and Briggs (1972) reported from it that those treated in the therapeutic community did better than those in a control group in terms of later recidivism but—perhaps more important—that in the four years of the project those who had been exposed to the latter two years, when the project was run largely by the offender group themselves, did better than those who took part in the initial two years, when there was a considerable staff involvement and influence. Developing from this recognition of the resources within the group itself, the *New Careers* project was set up at Vacaville and is described by Hodgkin (1972). In this, selected prisoners were not only involved in a therapeutic community programme but were also trained as social aides for a variety of social and rehabilitatory projects, particularly in the field of delinquency prevention, and a high success rate is reported following discharge from prison. A similar New Careers project is now in operation under the Borstal services at Bristol.

At Grendon Underwood in the UK, a psychiatric prison was opened in 1962 having first been suggested by Hubert and East in 1939. Gray (1974) reports on its general format and early results. With a population of 220 adult and young (Borstal) offenders, all male, the unit has experimented with a variety of treatments for what may be loosely termed 'psychopathic offenders'. The Borstal (young male offender) reconviction rate is the lowest for any closed Borstal, and in the boys' wing the re-conviction rate in the section that operates in a paternalistic authoritarian way is twice that in the therapeutic community-orientated section. Evaluation of the adult wing is more complex. It seems that short-term (under twelve months) treatment is of little effect but thereafter, the positive treatment effect rises. There is a complex interaction between group influence and time in treatment. Thus, those who come in on a group intake and stay only a short time do badly when compared with someone who comes in as an individual and is thus not subjected to group influence. The group influence thus seems to weigh against success initially. In the long term, however, those who come in with a group and stay over a year do better than those who come in as individuals. There is, thus, a positive attitude change by the group as time passes. This counter-culture of the prison world however was noted to be a prime factor in the failure of a therapeutic community regime in a Canadian prison by Fisher (1968). Offenders were unable to develop a degree of trust in the system or assume a peer group responsibility. The effect on the staff was to make them press harder for results, thus increasing the staff and inmate distance. Wilfert (1971) has described how essential it is to develop a horizontal authority structure in a penal therapeutic community rather than the traditional vertical one and to implement group-centred decision-making. An enquiry by Marcus (1969) at Grendon demonstrated a high allegiance of the prison officers to the therapeutic community system with less inmate–officer distance than is customary in a prison and also less officer–(professional) therapist distance, with the majority favourable to the treatment philosophy. Clearly this positive climate of therapy is important for success.

In approved schools, Jones (1973) made a study of different attitudes and regimes and the differing responses to them of the inmates. Thus, a school that stressed a disciplined approach produced boys unable to make peer relationships. In a less disciplined and more liberal school such relationships developed but the boys were just as aggressive as in the former. In a very repressive school there were no positive personality changes to report but in a 'progressive' school there was considerable expression of opinion and feeling but little or no positive change in behaviour.

He stresses that there is no 'best method' for universal application but some matching of the individual to the regime is necessary.

Group counselling or group psychotherapy, in prisons as distinct from an overall therapeutic community approach has also been described. Deane (1972) reports on group discussions related to reality problems as being most effective in promoting self-help, e.g. in the problems to be faced with discharge. Lenneer–Axelson (1969) is just one who describes the initial aggressive, hostile and suspicious opening to groups conducted in a prison setting, later to be replaced by expressions of loneliness and isolation and a feeling of alienation from other social groupings even after discharge, so that considerable after-care support is necessary.

Group work in the Probation Service is reviewed in a Home Office publication (1966). While a quarter of all probation areas were using groups at that time, only a few officers and a minority of clients were involved. The groups were broadly either discussions or activities, and deeper psychotherapy with the more disturbed clients was avoided. In the discussion groups the members themselves were seen as giving most support and control, while in the activity groups the officers took over these roles. Although three-quarters of these officers using groups felt that they were successful, the majority used them in combination with individual methods.

Again it is reported that evaluation is difficult. For instance, O'Brien (1961) actually showed that male juvenile offenders treated in groups scored worse on tests of socialisation and responsibility—but they had become more open and self-disclosing. Mays (1959) describes two types of groups for offenders: the psychologically orientated discussion group for those with emotional problems and the more socially orientated activity group for those with disorders rooted more in social disturbance.

The conclusion of this Home Office report is that there is encouraging evidence of change attributable to group therapies with probationers but as yet no proof of benefit.

The final word must go to the encyclopaedic review of Lipton et al. (1975). They collected and reviewed the papers published throughout the world from 1945 to 1967 on offender therapy.

Only studies that met stringent criteria of sound methodology, control comparison and reliable evaluation were considered. The results are somewhat difficult to summarise, nevertheless.

On recidivism, group counselling was found to be ineffective with male young offenders of fifteen to seventeen years (Seckel 1965). With adult offenders group counselling produced mixed results, but when a reduction in recidivism was found it was slight and the antagonistic negative effect of the prison culture is also remarked upon. Group psychotherapy in penal institutions was shown to be effective in reducing recidivism in males of fifteen to nineteen years (Persons and Pepinsky, 1966) but not with psychopaths of low intelligence (Craft et al., 1964), who became more recidivist than the control group treated in a benignly authoritarian way. Truax et al. (1966), using a Rogerian client-centred group approach, showed an improvement with institutionalised young females, and Taylor (1967), working in a New Zealand Borstal for girls, demonstrated that although no overall reduction in reconvictions was achieved girls treated by group psychotherapy were reconvicted of less serious offences and showed marked psychological improvement compared with girls treated by group counselling or routine care.

To summarise the summaries from Lipton *et al.* (1975), we can say that group psychotherapy is more effective than group counselling, although neither produces marked amelioration in recidivism. Group psychotherapy, however, has the potential for releasing increasingly disturbed emotional behaviour which requires skilled and knowledgable handling to turn to beneficial effect, and in this respect group work with young females seems more promising than with young males.

Perhaps the outstanding feature of all of these studies of various group methods on socially deviant individuals is that different regimes, in terms of the amount of external control, peer group support or self-responsibility that they employ, produce different effects on the individuals exposed to them depending on the degree of social maturity and personality functioning of the individual, and that what is essential from the outset is a correct assessment of the needs that can then be met with an appropriate treatment regime.

The family as a group in treatment

Perhaps no more challenging yet practical use of the group setting in psychiatric treatment has been made than in the field of family therapy.

In the 1950s various investigators were looking at disturbance of the family as a whole as a causative agent in the mental illness of one family member. The first explorations were in schizophrenia, but this work was later extended to the general misperceptions, mal-communications, confusing messages and role deficiencies that occur between members of a family living intimately together.

In the 1960s techniques of family therapy were developed based on psychoanalytic and on sociological theories or combinations of the two, but in actual practice the approaches had much in common (Stein, 1969).

Murray Bowen (1966) observed that 'the family is a system in that change in one part of the system is followed by compensatory change in other parts'. He drew attention to the *overadequate–inadequate* reciprocity that occurs between members with one member over-compensating for the dysfunction of another, and to the *emotional divorce* between the parents of a schizophrenic child with each maintaining a calm controlled distance, unable to communicate thoughts or feelings except perhaps to others outside the family circle. The child is then involved in an interdependent triad, becoming disturbed when the parents 'divorce' and do not communicate directly with each other but only to or through the child, and improving when direct communication between the parents was resumed. Bowen also described the *undifferentiated family ego mass*, which holds the family members together in an emotional interaction in a deeper way than the more transactional interactions between the members of an ordinary 'stranger' group. For Bowen, as for Beels and Ferber (1969), who review the various objectives of family therapy, the goal is to change the family system of interaction and, while families initially present with the sick member, it is the first task of the therapist to get the family to accept that the total family system must change. The therapist becomes the 'consultant', supervising the family in their exploration of the family problem and its resolution. Other investigators of this period drew attention to the *alignments and splits* that occur between family members (Wynne, 1962) and the *marital schism* (Lidz *et al.*, 1957) in the parents of schizophrenics, with the partners disunited and competing for the child's loyalty. Finally, Jackson (1957) drew attention to the *family homeostasis* and the upset occurring in other family members when the sick member improved.

The Palo Alto Medical Research Foundation was also looking at family interactions in the 1950s and Bateson (Bateson *et al.*, 1956) and others formulated the concept of the *'double-bind'*, wherein one member (usually the parent) gave a verbal message to another (usually the child) but simultaneously contradicted the message by non-verbal communication or inference; e.g. 'We love you and want you, of course—and we hope you will soon be well enough to leave home and live an independent life.' Virginia Satir (1967) expands the double-bind into the *denotative content* (what is literally said) and the *meta-communication* (the affective component), which asks a question and also implies what the answer should be; e.g. 'Well—we know that *we* love *you* . . .' (but do *you* love *us*?—because that is what you should be saying). Directness of communication is therefore necessary to maintain levels of understanding, and Satir believes that improved communication is the nub of family treatment and that the therapist must be a model for this.

The role of the therapist is described by Beels and Ferber (1969), who distinguish the conductors from the reactors. *Conductors* play a more dominant role, entering the family group to lead it by example (Satir, 1967), teaching and exploration. Minuchin *et al.* (1967), for instance, actually separate off from the family a member or members who are over-involved in a dispute or conflict between the remaining members and have them watch the interaction of the latter through a one-way screen showing them what is going on. The emphasis in Minuchin's group interventions is to break up established and dysfunctional methods of interaction and substitute new ones.

Paul (1967) explores in the family group the three-tier generational system, pointing out directly to a wife, perhaps, that she is being expected to fill the role of the lost mother for the grieving husband while the child is jealously dismissed. Bell (1961) proceeds phase by phase through exploration of the child's situation and how others see it to the child–parent situation, and thence to the marital situation.

The *reactors* are those therapists who respond to the family needs in a more psychoanalytic and transferential way, sometimes being central to the arguments and at other times peripheral. They tend to utilise co-therapists—male and female teams—to handle the mother and father transference and role situations. Whitaker (1965) describes almost an acting-out role for the therapist who sides with one or other member to activate the conflict situation and highlight the interaction. Zuk (1967) takes the activation even further, seeing the manipulation of power as the central issue and resorting to tricks in order to defeat the defensive efforts of the family. He will tell a rowing couple to 'go home and have a quarrel tonight', to which they will silently respond 'why should we do as he wishes?' and harmony reigns.

While the psychoanalysts have contributed to family therapy, the giving of insights through interpretation appears secondary to the enactment of the reality situation and the exploration of new channels of behaviour for most family therapists. Instead of asking, 'why do you think mother does not talk to you?' the therapists says 'see if you can get mother to talk to you, now'. The family therapist is more active, more direct, more intimate and more personally reactive than the conventional group therapist. He provides, however, an element of external control which allows the family to release their considerable pent-up emotions about each other, and, according to Skynner and to others, without any great calamity occurring in what at first might seem a fraught area.

Skynner (1969) gives us a very practical guide to the group-analytic treatment of the family. Both parents and all the children are expected to attend from the outset. Although Bell has suggested that children under nine be excluded because of their limited verbal communication, Skynner draws attention to the non-verbal interaction of and with the younger members. When a member of the family is repeatedly left at home the therapist may sometimes be cast in the role of this problem person and must be aware of the projections.

The time for each session is one-and-a-half hours and the general seating arrangement is a circle, but the one who sits aligned with or opposite to the therapist is worthy of note. The first session can usefully be employed as a mutual 'finding out' by taking a living history, as it were, from the family as a whole rather than coming to the meeting with a pre-written history and formulation from a social case-worker's reports. While the family tend to present the symptom as lodged in one member, Skynner draws the total family into the problem by asking what 'the symptom' is meant to communicate; what effect does 'the symptom' have on the rest of the family and, third, what the family interaction is to the symptom. Thus, in what is almost a role-playing situation, the family behaviour around the problem soon begins to emerge and can be commented upon as a family syndrome rather than as the ailment of one member. The frequency of sessions in this method is kept down to one every three weeks so that transference outside the family to the therapist is minimal and the family can work on their problem and the emerging insights in the intervals. Striking results are reported in 'one or two sessions and rarely as many as ten are needed', claims Skynner.

Two common dynamics in the family group are the concept of *boundaries* (Skynner, 1974) and the idea of the *family myth* (Byng–Hall, 1973). In the former the family is seen as more or less united within a boundary that sets it apart from the outside world. Within the bounds each member, too, has his own psychic boundaries of separateness from the others. Boundaries, however, can be tough and impenetrable or weak and diffuse, leading to defensive behaviour or to uncertainty and insecurity at the polar extremes. The problem child can be excluded from the family bounds by a family that is huddling together to deny the problem or, equally, can be possessively and defensively prevented from escaping over the family boundary. The therapist works at the boundary perhaps facilitating the re-entry of one or the freeing of another, as it seems appropriate.

The *family myth* refers to a situation first described by Ferreira (1963) as a family defence mechanism. The family members unconsciously collude in a defensive system of unreal and distorted roles which are unquestioned within the family and prevent exploration of the real family conflicts. Thus, the good-for-nothing son blames his inability to function on the overpowering matriarch. His wife agrees that the mother's interference prevents their marriage flourishing and the sisters too, unable to accept the uselessness of the males in the family, repose all power in the allegedly overbearing mother, who herself finds gratification in the concept since, this way at least, she maintains contact with her brood. In therapy the multiple projections are disentangled. This is done gently, as they are defensive mechanisms to protect each individual against more deeply felt inadequacies than is the relatively superficial 'family myth' which maintains a certain unsatisfactory homeostasis.

Crisis family therapy

Crisis intervention is a technique whereby, for instance, the request for hospitalisation for psychiatric treatment for one member of a family is met by an emergency home visit, usually by a psychiatrist, social worker and nurse. The goal of the crisis team is to explore the family network and detect the source of the disturbance that resulted in one member displaying sick symptoms. The whole family is summoned home for the conference and the ailment is centred on the family rather than the designated patient. Responsibility is put back on the family for creating the crisis situation, and resolution of the basic conflict is now sought within the family resources rather than by hospitalising the one who has broken down. In this way Pittman *et al.* (1966) at Colorado demonstrated that 84 per cent of referred cases could be kept out of hospital but, they state,

we did not delude ourselves that our method of crisis family therapy produces any personality pattern changes in the patient or even any permanent changes in the family. We hope we are discouraging chronicity, blunting some of the weapon value of symptoms and demonstrating to families that they can resolve crises more economically and function more gratifyingly.

Multiple family therapy groups

Treatment of three or four families together is a way of allowing both *family boundaries* to be broadened and *family myths* to be dissolved through shared experiences. Opportunities for empathy and learning from each other occur much as if each family were an individual meeting others in a group of individual strangers. The technique can have particular value, for instance, when the parents are gripped in a defensive and collusive pairing over the problem child. No movement takes place as long as they are seen alone or even as a whole family, but set alongside a parental couple or a family group with a similar problem, each member begins to interact with the opposite member of the other family in a way he is unable to operate with his own family member. The bottled-up father angrily denounces the other family's son; the repressed wife flirts a little with the other husband, and this acting through of other intrinsic problems can then be commented upon and brought back to the family or couple in which it resides by the therapist or the other group members.

Conjoint marital therapy

In conjoint marital therapy one couple only may be seen by the therapist but the danger of being cast in the role of referee can arise thereby. A group composed of three or four married couples gets over this hurdle and promotes the same opportunities for empathy, identification and relating to another couple's problems as is seen in multiple family therapy. Male and female co-therapists are of particular value in such a group and modelling on their behaviour and interaction is seen as an important treatment factor. In this respect some marital therapists are themselves married to each other and have reported on the beneficial influence this has on the group (Skynner *et al.*, 1975).

Hastings and Runkle (1963) report that in the early stages of such a group communications tend to be restricted to hostile comments from the more active partner to the passive and the *marriage neurosis*, as he terms it, is the main resistance to progress in treatment. As this is resolved the partners shift their objective to correcting their own emotional problems rather than seeking to correct the partner. The freeing of communication between the couples can be a major accomplishment, and this, too, is seen as the primary objective when a couple is seen as a dyad rather than in the group. Blocked communications between the partners, particularly over sexual difficulties, appears to be a common cause of silent or displaced hostility and can be rectified relatively quickly by a supportive and somewhat directive therapist (Skynner, 1975).

The evaluation of
group psychotherapy

The preceding chapters document the widespread clinical use of groups for purposes of personality change and behaviour modification. Many varieties of group work (small psychotherapy groups, encounter groups, T-groups, ward groups, large groups), a multiplicity of theoretical orientations (psychoanalytic, group-analytic, group-dynamic, therapeutic community) and a range of clients (in-patients, outpatients, delinquents, married couples, families) have al been mentioned. To conclude this survey, it is necessary to review some of the difficulties involved in carrying out psychotherapy research in general and to consider some theoretical issues, methods and empirical findings in evaluation studies of group techniques in particular.

The effectiveness of psychotherapy: problems of evaluation

Eysenck's (1952, 1960, 1965) conclusion that psychotherapy is ineffective, based on his reading of the evidence that about two-thirds of neurotic patients improve regardless of how, or even whether, they are treated, has been disputed but has also encouraged a greater concern for more evaluation in psychotherapy. (Malan, 1973, and Bergin, 1971, survey the specific arguments against Eysenck's handling of the data.) Eysenck's implicit assumptions that 'neurotic' patients were basically alike and that 'psychotherapy' as a generic entity could be evaluated are examples of what Kiesler (1971) has called uniformity myths. Researchers have vied with one another, attempting either to support Eysenck's position or to prove that 'psychotherapy' works. The complexities within and relationships between at least four salient variable groupings—patients, therapists, treatment theory and techniques and outcomes—were frequently not specified in published accounts; replication and comparison consequently becomes impossible, and results could be considered only suggestive at best. The search seemed to be for an elusive 'one best way', 'the *one system* of therapist behaviour that would produce constructive personality change for patients' (Kiesler, 1971).

Bergin (1971), after a thorough survey of outcome evaluations, frankly stated 'that gross tests of the effects of therapy are obsolete'. But he did not attribute the paucity of interpretable research to a pervasive operation of uniformity myths; rather, he stressed the methodological limitations and unreliability of measurement techniques, as well as the sheer complexity of the research enterprise. The investigations that Bergin surveyed revealed extreme variability of outcome no matter what the diagnosis, criteria of improvement or type of therapist. Many did not compare the experimental treatment with a control group of any kind, did not account for placebo (attention) effects which may be considerable in psychotherapy and so-called spontaneous remissions (cf. Shapiro, 1971, on placebo effects and Bergin, 1971, on spontaneous remission), or did not conduct adequate follow-up, all of which are fraught with tremendous difficulties. For example, Bergin pointed out that a true no-treatment control may be impossible to attain in that people are continually engaged in seeking out help when they are under strain and often find what can only be called therapeutic agents in a variety of extra-treatment settings. This consideration applies to the questions of spontaneous remissions and follow-up as well, for a scientific evaluation of both must include an assessment of potentially deteriorative and therapeutic intervening influences acting on treatment and control groups. The longer the follow-up, the more such influences can affect outcome and the more difficult it becomes to prevent the confounding of treatment with the passage of time, maturation or history. Bergin's advice to those who attempt to answer the question 'Does (or doesn't) psychotherapy work?' was 'that psychotherapy is such a heterogeneous collection of diverse and conflicting events that any attempt to definitely test its effect by virtue of classical pre-post control group designs is doomed to failure' (Bergin, 1971).

A number of other writers have added to the litany of complexities intrinsic to evaluation research and have made many fundamental recommendations (Strupp and Bergin, 1969; Strupp and Luborsky, 1962; Rubinstein and Parloff, 1959; Shlien *et al.*, 1968; Bergin and Garfield, 1971; Truax and Carckhuff, 1967; Meltzoff and Kornreich, 1970; Malan, 1959, 1973; Frank, 1961; G. L.

Paul, 1967). Researchers' attention is directed to the need to ensure homogeneous patient groups matched on relevant variables; to operationalise in specific therapist behaviour the concepts of particular theoretical perspectives; to recognise that a choice of change or outcome criteria implies a question of values; to assess theory-specific kinds, directions and magnitudes of change; to make predictions that are capable of being disproved; to understand in greater depth the natural history of specific mental illnesses and, in particular, the form (not necessarily monotonic) that change takes over time; to be aware that, since change is multidimensional, there may be low intercorrelations between various measures of change even when criteria are carefully selected in line with theoretical predictions; to evaluate concurrently therapy process and outcome, often artificially separated; and, following from the last point, to clearly specify and distinguish intra- and extra-therapy dependent variables and theoretically to link mediating variables with more superordinate treatment goals.

Evaluation methods in psychotherapy

In effect, many researchers have cast their questions in a totally different form. Paul (1967) asks, 'What treatment, by *whom*, is most effective for *this* individual with *that* specific problem, and under *which* set of circumstances ?' To answer this question in a scientifically meaningful way, Paul proposed the consideration of three major domains, cutting across theoretical orientation, which are involved in psychotherapy research. *Clients* must be characterised in terms of their problem behaviours, their relatively stable personal–social attributes and their physical–social life environment. *Therapists'* techniques and personal–social characteristics, as well as the treatment environment, must be distinguished. Finally, *time* must be analysed in terms of the duration of various stages (initial contact, pre-treatment, initial treatment, main treatment, termination, post-treatment and follow-up) and interactions with other variables.

Paul's main purpose is to provide a conceptual scheme to deal particularly with the problems of control, in order to help eliminate as much confounding of variables as possible. While case studies may provide the clinical researcher with crude hypotheses, confounding within and between all three domains is likely. Factorial group designs with no-treatment and placebo–attention controls are a far more rigorous method and afford causal explanations with no necessary confounding inherent in the design.

Such methodological classicism may be a desirable ideal to aim for in principle. In practice, single case studies, which can be quite rigorous (cf. Barlow and Hersen, 1973; Chassan, 1967) may be essential to help clarify the specifics implied by Paul's formulation of the proper research question. This approach is well suited to clinical practice, and requires systematic specification of disorders, interventions and changes over time with flexible modifications of technique until the desired effect is attained. Once regularities and patterns are observed, fruitful extension to nomothetic studies will be possible (Bergin, 1971). Another alternative, closer to Paul's paradigm, is the use of experimental analogues which, although conducted in a setting very different from the clinical one, permit stringent controls and may eventually generate suggestive hypotheses (Heller, 1971). Replication studies on patient populations would be a means of determining the relevance of laboratory experiments.

Kiesler, like Paul, emphasises the importance of asking specific research questions, and he conceptualises the issues in terms of a grid model (Kiesler, 1969, 1971). This model also requires the specification of homogeneous patient groups, based not so much on traditional nosological categories as on characteristics entailed by specific theories (i.e. hostility, dependency, oral character, need for approval); the specification of expected changes—symptomatic, behavioural, psychodynamic—required by the theory (for one patient the therapeutic aim might be to *increase* the anxiety level while another might need to show a diminution on this dimension if the treatment is to be considered effective); the specification of time and the interaction of time with both patient changes and therapist interventions or behaviours; and the specification of therapist interventions, personality characteristics (which may need to be matched with patients) and attitudes that theoretically correspond with specific changes in specific groups of patients. The overriding concern for Kiesler is that 'one casts the theoretical statements in a form leading to predictable consequences in the observable domain, and then sets up operations that can confirm or disconfirm these predictions' (Kiesler, 1971).

For Paul and Kiesler, no one study can 'evaluate psychotherapy', nor can it do more than contribute to a continuing accumulative research process. Factorial designs, which are very difficult to set up properly, are recommended by both. Malan (1963, 1976a,b) has utilised an alternative methodology, which, while considerably less complicated and more suitable to clinical conditions, realises the specificity approach advocated by other workers in the field. His main objective is to formulate '*outcome criteria that do justice to the complexity of the human personality*' (Malan, 1973). Since Malan's theoretical orientation is psychoanalytic, these criteria are psychodynamic, and are based on the principle used in the psychotherapy project of the Menninger Clinic that 'there is no substitute for a judgment made by an experienced clinician, properly applied' (quoted in Malan, 1973). The procedure is to list all the known disturbances in an individual's life; to make a psychodynamic hypothesis which links the disturbances; to specify in advance of follow-up the 'ideal' changes in each disturbance if the treatment were to be effective; to compare the actual changes with the predicted 'ideal'; and to rate the result on a scale. In his study of brief focal psychotherapy, Malan (1963) found that, once meaningful (in terms of theory and subtlety) outcome criteria were established individually for each patient, not only do positive therapeutic results occur but significant correlations with process variables also come to light.

However, Malan has cautioned that his design does not deal with the problem of spontaneous remissions, which may occur even among the treated cases. With his colleagues at the Tavistock Clinic he has conducted research into the natural history of untreated neurotic patients from a psychodynamic perspective (Malan, *et al.*, 1968, 1973). Few authors who have studied this issue accept without qualification Eysenck's spontaneous recovery figure of two-thirds. Bergin (1971), for example, believes the figure of 30 per cent would reflect a more accurate reading of the investigations on which Eysenck relied. Malan *et al.* found that spontaneous remission was less on dynamic criteria than on behavioural (30–50 per cent compared with 60–70 per cent) and concluded that 'this result casts some doubt on the statement that roughly two-thirds of neurotic patients "get better" without treatment' (Malan *et al.*, 1968). The resolution of this issue awaits more long-term follow-ups of both treated and untreated patients which should include a careful study of the total social environments in which they live (Moos, 1974). But it is clear that spontaneous remissions—and indeed reports of the effects of a particular treatment—vary according to the stringency of outcome criteria employed.

Deterioration effects

Before turning to consider some results of group psychotherapy evaluation studies, one additional crucial finding regarding outcome should be mentioned: the existence of deterioration or negative effects (Cartwright, 1956; Bergin, 1963, 1966, 1967a,b, 1970, 1971; Malan, 1973; Hadley and Strupp, 1976). Most evaluations cast the data in the form of comparisons between *average* outcome of the treatment group with either another treatment or a 'no-treatment' control. This obscures the fact that the variation or spread of outcome scores in the treated group is regularly larger than that of the control group scores. The implication of this finding is that psychotherapy is powerful, that it can make some people get worse and that other people show improvements far beyond those manifested by control subjects. By combining such different and opposing results to obtain a measure of average treatment efficacy, both significant improvements and significant deteriorations cancel one another out and show no advantage for the treatment compared with no treatment and spontaneous remission.

The demonstration of deterioration effects has confirmed a widespread conviction among practitioners that negative effects are common and even more frequent than clinicians like to admit. Hadley and Strupp (1976) have conducted a survey of expert opinion on this issue. They asked 150 clinicians, researchers and theoreticians if they believed that there was a problem of negative effects. In addition, respondents were requested to comment on the criteria they use to ascertain whether a patient has become worse as a direct result of psychotherapy and to specify the causative factors associated with negative effects.

The experts who replied (approximately 50 per cent) virtually unanimously believed 'that there is a real problem of negative effects in psychotherapy' (Hadley and Strupp, 1976). They mentioned several categories of negative effects which included such obvious manifestations as the exacerbation of presenting symptoms and the development of new symptoms. Other, more subtle, negative effects included the misuse/abuse of therapy by a patient, for example by substitution of psychological jargon for previous obsessional thoughts or over-emphasis on intra-psychic exploration to the detriment of constructive action outside of treatment; the undertaking of unrealistic tasks and goals which often leads to excessive strain and inevitable disappointment; and loss of trust in the therapist and psychotherapy, perhaps even in all relationships.

Among factors associated with negative effects, the respondents noted inaccurate or deficient assessment, ignorance and deficiencies in therapist training and personality characteristics, masochistic character structure and intense guilt reactions in patients, mis-applications or rigidities of technique, counter-transference problems and difficulties in patient–therapist communication. Of particular importance is the 'compendium' of mistakes in technique which Hadley and Strupp derived from the questionnaires. They call attention to omnipotent assumptions regarding the scope and efficacy of therapy, a failure to specify goals (intermediate and ultimate) that are realistic for the patient in question, the excessive focusing of therapy on insights and interpretations rather than 'behaviour and will', the mis-matching of therapy to the patient's disturbance, which may result in overly intense therapy in which premature interpretations shatter defences without providing an alternative source of support, and dependency-fostering techniques (therapy as addiction). In essence, these views and the research evidence on deterioration effects highlight the importance of evaluating evaluation studies themselves according to whether they are addressed to Bergin's question, which echoes Kiesler, Paul, Malan and others: 'What are the specific effects of specific inter-ventions by specified therapists upon specific symptoms or patient types ?' (Bergin, 1971).

Problems in evaluating group psychotherapy

The complexities and difficulties inherent in doing even individual psychotherapy research are daunting. A survey of group psycho-therapy evaluation studies reveals an exponential increase in both complexity and difficulty as well as a corresponding decrease in rigorous and interpretable investigations. The scientific ideal of control becomes more elusive in the face of group processes and spontaneous, multi-person interactions.

Burchard et al. (1948) remarked on the lack of any systematic collection and analysis of data. Kotkov (1956) noted that only approximately 2 per cent of the group psychotherapy research papers that he had seen were experimental. Slavson (1962) com-mented on the deficient use of objective methods in outcome research. Pattison (1965) found that, in six major volumes on psychotherapy research published during the ten-year period 1956–66, fewer than six references were made to evaluation studies. In Meltzoff and Kornreich's (1970) monumental review of the psychotherapy research literature—Malan (1973) called it 'the review to end all reviews'—only 7 per cent of the references were to group therapy. Frank (1975) surveyed at random ten issues published between 1955 and 1973 of the *International Journal of Group Psychotherapy* and discovered that only 7.5 per cent of all papers, i.e. thirty-eight papers, were devoted to research. One-half concerned outcome and the rest were process studies or miscellaneous topics such as investigations of selection, attendance and drop-outs. 'Only two address the research question probably most relevant to practice, which is the relationship of process and aspects of process to outcome' (Frank, 1975).

The *International Journal of Group Psychotherapy* publishes an annual review of the group psychotherapy literature and for the most part the various authors confirm Frank's comment. Lubin *et al.* (1972) reported that a greater proportion of the articles they reviewed were 'research based', although virtually all of this research was process studies. Reddy and Lansky (1974) found that many studies remained descriptive or anecdotal and 'as in the past, there is a dearth of carefully designed and executed research.' Reddy *et al.* (1975) were pleased that relatively brief group experiences, which are more amenable to investigation, were the focus of increasing attention, but they admitted that 'although there are substantial research efforts, relatively thorough and extensive research projects or those which focus on long-term follow-up assessment are little in evidence' (Reddy *et al.*, 1975). In 1975 the *Journal* marked its twenty-fifth anniversary, and the same authors stated that 'the criticisms of the past must be made again: minimal programmatic research, overstatement of anecdotal findings, studies ill-conceived and poorly controlled . . . because of limitations in methodology many findings can only be viewed with suspicion as being of questionable reliability and validity' (Reddy *et al.*, 1976).

Summarising a group psychotherapy research pnael conducted under the auspices of the *International Journal of Group Psychotherapy* Parloff wrote that in his view 'anyone who undertakes to review group psychotherapy process and outcome studies has already undergone strange and unnatural punishment' (Parloff, 1967). He went on to repeat many of the same points regarding methodological deficiencies that have been discussed above, and speculated that perhaps researchers were trapped by a repetition compulsion which masked an underlying defensiveness regarding their uncertainties and doubts as to the effectiveness of psychotherapy:

> Since the selected studies do not apparently provide adequate information regarding the 'kinds' of patients, the nature of psychotherapy, or the criteria and measures of outcome employed, it is difficult to compare these studies or to become aware of meaningful interactions among the variables cited. . . . The research papers continue to be inadequate, and reviewers persist in going through the exercise of reviewing essentially trivial reports.

Parloff was extremely concerned that he had held such a critical and pessimistic view for over twenty years and he warned that 'unless our tolerance for what we choose to call ambiguity is sharply lessened, the entire field of group psychotherapy may assume the unhappy stature of being the Peter Pan of psychotherapies' (Parloff, 1967).

Methods in the evaluation of group psychotherapy

In response to the 'flight from outcome into process' (Hoch and Zubin, 1964), Parloff (1970a) reiterated for group psychotherapy researchers the need to link a multiplicity of process variables, including therapist behaviours, with specific—and equally multidimensional—outcome criteria. The main weakness in most process studies was an unwarranted assumption of a 'simple relationship between all measures of the therapeutic relationship and all measures of outcome' (Parloff, 1970a). In a study of group psychotherapy dropouts, Parloff (1961) himself had exploded this particular 'uniformity myth'. He found that, when patients were rank-ordered in terms of the quality of the therapeutic relationship established in the group, the *relative* rather than the absolute quality of the relationship might be more important.

Parloff (1970a) also presented a model of outcome criteria which included two dimensions, *patient state* and *patient level*. Patient state describes two categories. The *affective state* refers to an individual's subjective experience and feeling, ranging from pain to pleasure and from dysphoria to euphoria. The *effective state* refers to behaviour that is observable, objective and can be evaluated on a scale ranging from ineffective, irresponsible and unproductive to effective, responsible and creative. The patient level is divided into the two categories of *headshrinking* and *mind-expanding*. Headshrinking refers to a spectrum of behaviour, feeling and experience ranging from extremely negative states to a 'hypothetical neutral or zero point' (Parloff, 1970a). Mind-expanding ranges from the neutral point through increasingly positive experiences, feelings and performances, i.e. peak states. Each level is analysed in terms of each state, and Parloff cautions against the assumption that simultaneous affective and effective changes will necessarily occur. In a subsequent discussion of 'Some Current Issues of Group Psychotherapy Research', Parloff (1973) insisted that no intermediate process criteria—such as Lewis and McCant's (1973) emphasis on change in the individual's relationships within the group—could be substituted for the ultimate goal, 'that the problems for which the patient sought help will, in fact, be ameliorated' (Parloff, 1973).

Pattison (1965) traced the historical development of evaluation and reviewed ninety studies of group psychotherapy. He pointed out the widespread omission of patient variables, the poor definition of therapeutic orientations and methods and the extreme heterogeneity of populations and outcome criteria—all of which made comparisons almost meaningless. Research on group psychotherapy, he suggested, 'involves a necessary distinction between group process and therapeutic process, between the effect of the therapist and that of the group, and between the outcome of the group and that of the person' (Pattison, 1965). Pattison emphasised the need to dissect each variable of the group psychotherapy enterprise, and he distinguished patients, types of therapy (techniques and theoretical position), context of therapy and therapy time (frequency and group phase). Finally, he recommended the conceptual clarification of variables along three continuua:

(1) *patients*—from the most primitive and severely regressed to out-patients functioning at the highest levels;
(2) *treatment techniques*—from regressive modes such as occupational, music and recreation therapy to those requiring more ego involvement such as ward meetings and milieu activities with increasing reliance on verbalization, insight and psychotherapy; and
(3) *treatment goals*—from status changes such as institutional

discharge or transfer to a less restrictive ward to basic behavioural changes, symptom alleviation, alterations in interpersonal activities, values and overall personal and social adjustment.

Different levels of patients have different problems and different techniques with different goals and measures of outcome. At the higher levels of each continuum, research tends to run out (Gundlach, 1967). Whatever the criteria, the two central questions are whether the measure reflects therapeutic change and not just change alone, and whether the measure reflects a unique group effect (Pattison, 1965).

Some results of group psychotherapy

General findings

Fully aware of all the difficulties, complexities, inadequacies and cautions surrounding the research endeavour, we conclude by presenting a representative sample of the kinds of results that are being reported in reviews of the evaluation literature and in particular investigations.

Bednar and Lawlis (1971) conducted a thorough analysis of empirical research in group psychotherapy. Their review of forty-nine evaluations spans a wide range of patients and techniques and includes research designs of varying rigour. It is particularly helpful in that the methodological problems specific to group psychotherapy *outcome* and *process* studies are discussed in detail. The authors also present data that confirm that deterioration effects occur in group psychotherapy.

Among Bednar and Lawlis's most important conclusions for both outcome and process are the following.

Outcome

(1) Group psychotherapy is a 'two-edged sword' and can help as well as harm patients. Therapists should seek systematic feed-back regarding their general effectiveness and the types of patients and group composition with which they are most and least able to work. Selection of patients is of crucial importance.

(2) Patients who are not easily able to verbalise and communicate feelings may benefit from pre-therapy training. The purpose of

such training would be to clarify role expectations, answer questions, provide information about the therapy process and generally orient the patient in preparation for a new experience.

(3) 'Group therapy has been reported effective with neurotics, psychotics, and patients with character disorders, with the most positive results being reported on neurotic symptomology [*sic*]. . . . The evidence is sufficiently clear to indicate the potential value of group therapy, irrespective of the treatment population, in any programme involved with institutional living' (Bednar and Lawlis, 1971).

(4) The first six post-treatment months are critical. Without follow-up contact which facilitates the transfer of new behaviours and insights, improvements reported at termination tend to dissipate over time.

Process

(1) Empirical evidence from group psychotherapy research corroborates the group-dynamic literature, which emphasises the significance of group cohesion. 'The cohesive atmosphere of the group is a primary antecedent to constructive personality change.' Well developed groups should be maintained not only throughout the successive phases of treatment but, if possible, during the difficult period of community readjustment. Criteria for determining compatible groups should be used in selection procedures.

This finding gives strong encouragement to researchers and practitioners such as Goldstein (1966; Goldstein and Simonson, 1971) Frank (1957), Durkin (1957) and Schneider (1955) who, among others, argue for the extrapolation and testing of group dynamics research in psychotherapy groups. This position does not assert the identity of all types of groups. Rather, as Parloff writes (quoted in Goldstein and Simonson, 1971):

> The fact that therapy groups differ in many ways from the training group or the problem-solving group on which the findings of group dynamics are based is not the crucial issue. The ultimate question is whether hypotheses regarding the inter-relationships among the variables in one set of groups are supported in . . . therapy groups.

(2) Silence, by itself, does not indicate emotional uninvolvement with the group and has not been empirically related to outcome. Involvement, on the other hand, is the critical variable.

(3) Groups with schizophrenic patients must be more structured initially with greater emphasis on activity level. Tasks, physical movement and the use of drugs may help to activate patient behaviour and alleviate the tensions arising from interpersonal relationships in the group.

(4) The presence of a group leader helps to maintain concentration on the therapeutic work. Leaderless groups may be more spontaneous and play-oriented.

Specific results

Positive results have consistently been reported by the Rogerian client–centred school (Truax and Carckhuff, 1967; Truax and Mitchell, 1971). The research basically deals with the therapist's interpersonal skills and attempts to identify certain 'prepotent therapist qualities' which cut across techniques and theories of psychotherapy and which can be related to process and outcome. The essential finding is that high levels of *accurate empathy*, *non-possessive warmth*, and *genuineness* provided by the therapist correlate with many measures of improvement including raters' judgements, MMPI, Q-sort, the Welsh Anxiety Index and time spent out of hospital during a one-year follow-up period. As a corollary, low levels of the conditions correlate with patient deterioration. Truax and Mitchell (1971) offer as an explanation the principle of 'reciprocal effect'. If the stimulus is a positive effect (i.e. high levels of the three therapist conditions), the patient's response will be in proportion and kind. High levels reinforce a positive self-concept, encourage deeper self-revelation in the group, diminish anxiety and promote human relating. The authors believe that their work supports the widely held assumption that a relationship exists between self-acceptance and acceptance of others.

An important implication of this generally optimistic work should be noted. Spontaneous remission is possibly a result of everyday contacts with what Truax and Mitchell call 'inherently helpful persons' who are able to offer high levels of the therapeutic conditions. Evidence adduced by them (1971) indicates that, at least for client-centred therapy, on *average* trained personnel have no more effect on outcome than do no treatment, untrained or briefly trained non-professionals. For the former,

> the odds are two out of three that he is spending his energy,
> commitment, and care for mankind wastefully; he is either

ineffective or harmful . . . Basically the personality of the therapist is more important than his techniques, although techniques can be powerful when allied with high conditions.

Shapiro (1976) has reviewed the data on which Truax and others (Truax and Carckhuff, 1967; Truax and Mitchell, 1971) based their positive results, and he commented that while the controlled studies do show moderately promising results, the correlational studies demonstrate only a weak association between levels of conditions and outcome. Many of the studies failed to control for differences in patients and for interaction effects between patients and therapists, and are criticised for being insufficiently experimental. Shapiro admits that 'one must recognise the great difficulty in furnishing conclusive scientific validation for any psychological treatment'. Bergin and Suinn (1975) reviewed much unpublished work and expressed scepticism as to the potency of the three conditions outside of a client-centred framework. In fact, Bergin (1971) considers the conditions to be prerequisites for any meaningful human relationship, i.e. non-specific to therapy. Bergin's view is not disputed by Truax and Mitchell, who wished to stress 'the commonality that psychotherapy has with other aspects of life' (Truax and Mitchell, 1971).

Sethna and Harrington (1971) conducted an evaluation of group psychotherapy with fifty-three in-patients and day-patients at a unit that deals primarily with neurotic and personality disorders. Thirty-five patients had analytic group psychotherapy only, while eighteen were treated with a combination of supportive group psychotherapy and drugs. The study is notable for the scope and relevance of its aims, which were to see (1) how patients' assessments of improvement or lack of it compared with the therapists' and researchers' observations; (2) how expectations of improvement compared with actual results; (3) how suitability for the group (on the basis of age, intelligence, anxiety level, motivation, secondary gains, ego strength and reality difficulties) related to sophistication in the group (awareness of group phenomena and processes) and outcome (relief of symptoms, improvement in interpersonal functioning, ability to cope with and adapt to a variety of life experiences, self-awareness and personality change); and (4) how much relative importance was attached to other treatment modalities.

The main result of this investigation was that suitability ratings predicted sophistication in the group as well as outcome. Younger patients (under forty) with moderate anxiety and expectations, fewer reality difficulties, higher intelligence, greater ego strength and motivation and less secondary gain remained in treatment longer, had less physical treatment, preferred group psychotherapy and improved the most. Therapists' ratings of outcome tended to be lower than patients', perhaps because the latter overemphasised relief of symptoms to the exclusion of other relevant criteria. Cabral and Paton (1975) reported a similar finding in their study of correlations between patients' and observers' rankings of outcome criteria.

Once again, the investigation of Sethna and Harrington highlights the critical nature of selection. Garfield's (1971) comprehensive review of the literature on patient variables associated with outcome revealed that intelligence, and social class with which it is interrelated, are strongly related to improvement. Personality inventories and projective tests, on the other hand, are of dubious predictive value. Caine and Wijesinghe (1976) have, however, developed a number of measures of personality and expectancies which they believe discriminate between patients who do well in group psychotherapy as compared with behaviour therapy. Their evidence shows, for example, that patients who subsequently do well in group psychotherapy will tend to hold particular pre-treatment attitudes. They will have confidence in the ability of other patients to help, will depend less on the doctor, will stress their symptoms less, will recognise interpersonal difficulties and will admit a need to change. In other words, they are psychologically rather than physically orientated. Correlated with these attitudes is a 'liberal' approach to social issues in general and a Jungian 'inward' direction of interest. Frank (1961, 1968) Goldstein (1962) and Goldstein et al. (1966) have clearly analysed the important complex relationship between expectations and both therapy process and outcome.

Sethna and Harrington (1971) concluded that their results 'were modest—but worthwhile' and that 'in the absence of more effective methods of treatment the use of group psychotherapy seems justified'.

Bovill (1972) designed a comparison of the relative effectiveness of treating initially hospitalised female neurotics with group psychotherapy and relaxation or the currently used routine methods which included individual interviews and electroplexy. The mean time in treatment was two sessions a week over thirty months and follow-up was one year when possible. Group psychotherapy was didactic and took the form of each patient in turn presenting a topic for discussion, usually a symptom or problem. Members of the control treatment $(N=36)$ were referred to out-patient clinics on discharge if they desired, while the group psychotherapy patients $(N=36)$ could continue in an open group for as long as they wanted after leaving hospital. The main outcome criterion was independence of the hospital, i.e. the capacity of the patient to remain at home. In addition, a questionnaire assessing symptoms, behaviour, work and general adjustment was prepared. Family doctors were contacted to determine the amount of attention and medication the patients needed. The results were overwhelmingly in favour of the group treatment. For every one day of subsequent rehospitalisation of a patient who had been involved in group psychotherapy, the control patient spent seven days. The well-being assessments were also significantly favourable. 'It was concluded that a consistent course of group psychotherapy and relaxation is beneficial to neurotic patients and that this is not uneconomical in doctors' time' (Bovill, 1972).

Dick (1975) treated ninety-three neurotic or borderline out-patients with group-analytic psychotherapy. Selection involved five preliminary individual psychotherapy sessions with a view to the appropriate matching of patient and treatment. The average time in treatment was sixty-three sessions over eighteen months. Three follow-ups were carried out with predictably shrinking response rates: 53 patients at six months, 45 at eighteen months and 44 at two and a half years. Outcome measures were similar to those used in the Sethna and Harrington study and included marital or patient–parent relationship, work, sex, physical health, leisure, self-image, self-understanding and symptoms. The result of this investigation was that 87 per cent of the patients showed a positive change, a few showed negative change and one became temporarily psychotic. Dick wrote that 'the majority appear to have been enabled to become independent of the psychiatric service and to become involved in a process of change'.

Similar very encouraging results can be found in the literature. Of particular interest are a number of studies of group process and of both intra- and inter-personal changes which use *repertory grid* methods. Since Kelly (1955) formulated his psychology of personal constructs and Bannister, primarily with his co-workers Mair

(Bannister and Mair, 1968) and Fransella (Bannister and Fransella, 1971) developed and popularised the theory, the repertory grid has been widely used by clinicians and researchers. Smail (1972) used the grid to study empathy between members and between members and therapists in a small therapeutic group. In effect, this research attempted to operationalise and measure one of the three crucial interpersonal skills singled out by Rogers (1957) and by Truax and Carckhuff (1967) and Truax and Mitchell (1971). Smail found positive relationships between empathy scores, on the one hand, and the kinds of attitudes (i.e. psychotherapeutic v. organic orientation) which he, Caine and Wijesinghe believe are important in selection and outcome (cf. Caine and Smail, 1969; Caine and Wijesinghe, 1976). Smail writes: 'It seems quite reasonable that the "psychologically minded" person, accustomed to thinking in terms of mental-subjective rather than physical-objective values . . . should be better at assessing correctly the mental operations of others.' Another possible interpretation of this evidence is that part of the relationship which has been found between 'psychological mindedness' and favourable outcome in group psychotherapy may be attributable to the fact that group members can empathise with and understand more deeply people who hold certain attitudes. This work may be illustrating an important interaction between group process (i.e. patterns of empathy) and personality types. Also concerned with the study of process, Fransella (1970) and Fransella and Joyston–Bechal (1971) have demonstrated with the repertory grid the group-determined nature of some of the changes that occur in what group members think about as well as in the way they think. The implication of these investigations is that a quantitative measure of cognitive and emotional content and form, related to group development over time, is feasible and may be related to outcome.

Another extremely productive type of repertory grid study is directed towards the explication of psychodynamic and inter-personal changes that take place in group psychotherapy. Ryle (1975) and his colleagues have used the grid in a variety of clinical contexts including small groups, conjoint marital therapy, group work with maladjusted couples and group treatment of students with emotional and learning difficulties. Ryle has recognised many of the complexities involved in the evaluation of group psycho-therapy, and in his paper with Lipshitz (Ryle and Lipshitz, 1976) found that most patients improved on some criteria but not on all.

He confirmed the low intercorrelations that other researchers have reported between different outcome indices and emphasised that only a rigorous, individualised approach to research could fully elicit the subtleties of changes.

Watson (1970, 1972) has illustrated the wide range of information tapped by the repertory grid methodology. When applied to the study of groups, the technique affords insight into the interpersonal relationships between the members, psychological processes of individuals and changes that occur over time. For example, by inspection of a grid in which each member including the therapist(s) rates himself, all the others and the group itself on a number of dimensions describing behaviour and feelings, one can determine the extent to which group members agree on how they see one another. In effect, this is a kind of sociogram. Mean ratings on the dimensions give some idea of how intensely or indifferently individuals or the group are being perceived. Correlations between dimensions, between elements (the entities being rated) and between dimensions and elements measure inferred psychological relationships. For one member, everyone rated highly on 'depressed' may also be so rated on 'angry', and one could hypothesise a psychological link between these two feelings for that person. Likewise, correlations between two people (elements) may be a measure of identification; i.e., 'I see myself as being like Joe' is inferred from similar ratings for both on most dimensions. Comparison of a series of grids provides a measure of changes in psychodynamic and interpersonal terms; e.g., identification between a man and his therapist, operationalised as a high positive correlation between 'self' and 'therapist' elements, may be seen to increase or decrease over time. The content of the dimensions on which 'self' and 'therapist' are rated may reveal some of the reasons for such changes; i.e., as 'therapist' becomes more 'admirable', identification perhaps increases. Watson's work is clearly significant in suggesting ways to explore the relationship between co-therapists, the relative importance of different group members, the emotional tone of the group, self-esteem and identifications and more complicated psychological mechanisms in single patients.

Unpublished data from a grid study of the experience of Henderson residents confirm that meaningful, dramatic changes result from intensive involvement in group treatment (Gordon, 1976). For example, the patient quoted in chapter 5 whose letter conveyed his own sense of the important changes that had occurred in his relationships to his wife and family completed a series of three grids at three-month intervals during treatment. The first, at admission, showed that he viewed his wife and mother as virtually identical in all ways, predominantly negative. He also saw himself as disliking and very unlike his father (i.e., low 'self'–'father' correlation). By the end of treatment, these grid measures were substantially altered. He could discriminate between his wife and mother and showed a more favourable and accepting insight into his father, with whom he recognised both positive and negative similarities.

Phillipson (1958) wrote of his evaluation of group treatment with psychoneurotic patients that

> in a large proportion of the severely disturbed cases well-evidenced progress is recorded. In many other cases attendance at the groups appears to have helped such very ill patients to continue to function, though still in an impaired fashion in the key areas of their lives.

Most of these studies can be criticised, and often the research designs employed are very weak, but many clinicians are reporting favourably on a range of group methods.

On the other hand, there is no lack of null results. Freeman's (1967) survey of 95 psychoneurotics showed that only 9 recovered, 20 improved and 66 did not change. Patients with a long history were significantly less improved, and none of the recovered patients had undergone previous treatment or hospitalisation, nor were they dependent on medication. Failure to improve was significantly associated with such dependence. In the no-change group, 52 per cent were from social classes IV and V while only 14 per cent of the other two outcome categories were in these classes. None of the recovered attended the group for less than one year and 58 per cent of the no-change patients attended for under six months. Freeman noted the self-selection process occurring over time and, given the 'dismal results', considered group psychotherapy 'too expensive a procedure for routine employment' in the NHS. He cautioned that 'the experience of the group experiment shows, however, that a selection procedure is absolutely essential if psychotherapy resources are to be appropriately and correctly deployed' (Freeman, 1967). Incidentally, this study found fairly positive results for individual psychotherapy.

Finally, Malan *et al.* (1976) investigated 'the effectiveness of *insight-orientated group psychotherapy with adult psychoneurotic out-patients*'. Their review of the sparse number of controlled studies on this topic led to the verdict: 'The results are not impressive.' The positive results of group therapy at termination either dissipated with time or were inferior to de-sensitization. Malan and his colleagues also considered the studies by Freeman, Phillipson and Sethna and Harrington, and they justifiably wrote that these investigations 'show a wide spectrum in their conclusions about the effectiveness of group treatment'.

Although Malan's study is retrospective and of necessity used short-stay patients as controls, the design did control for the passage of time, follow-up was unusually long (two to fourteen years) and the psychodynamic outcome criteria were rigorously formulated. The sample size was quite small (forty-two randomly selected patients and thirteen 'stars', i.e. patients selected by their therapists for particularly notable improvement). The result of this carefully conceived project was summarised by the authors as follows (Malan *et al.*, 1976)

> Comparison of psychodynamic changes in patients who stayed
> more than two years gave a null result. The majority
> of patients were highly dissatisfied with their group
> experiences. However, there was a very strong positive
> correlation between favourable outcome and *previous
> individual psychotherapy*.

The star cases had also certainly improved, but whether such change was specifically a group effect remained an open question despite some clinical evidence (interviews) that some of these patients did attribute their progress to the group experience. The authors recommend that particular attention be directed to the crucial phases of selection, preparation for therapy, termination and follow-up contacts.

Referring to their survey of a multiplicity of techniques of verbal therapy with many types of patient, Meltzoff and Kornreich (1970) summarised:

> In short, reviews of the literature that have concluded that
> psychotherapy has, on average, no demonstrable effect are
> based upon an incomplete survey of the existing body of
> research and an insufficiently stringent appraisal of the data.

We have encountered no comprehensive review of controlled research on the effects of psychotherapy that has led convincingly to a conclusion in support of the null hypothesis. ... In general, the better the quality of the research, the more positive the results obtained [quoted in Malan, 1973].

Clearly, the unequivocal application of this judgement to methods of group psychotherapy would be premature. While the published results of outcome studies of group psychotherapy on average show only modest improvement in terms of behaviour change, it is evident that the process of psychotherapy in the group is a powerful dynamic which seldom has little or no effect on the individuals taking part. The interaction of the group process with the particular personalities of the group members provokes and releases psychological and interpersonal forces of a high order.

Whether it is just to be aware of the dynamic forces of the milieu or to utilise the group process as a positive change agent, a highly skilled and sensitive approach is required, towards which we hope this book will serve as a useful guide.

A basic library of books on group treatments in psychiatry

BERNE, E., *Principles of Group Treatment*, Oxford University Press, New York, 1966.

BION, W. R., *Experiences in Groups*. Tavistock, London, 1961.

CARTWRIGHT, D. and ZANDER, A., *Group Dynamics. Research and Theory*, Tavistock, London, 1968.

FOULKES, S. H., *Group Analytic Psychotherapy: Method and Principles*, Gordon & Breach, London, 1975.

FREUD, S., *Group Psychology and the Analysis of the Ego*, Hogarth Press, London, 1921; re-issued 1967.

KREEGER, L. (ed.), *The Large Group*, Constable, London, 1975.

LIEBERMAN, M. A., YALOM, I. D. and MILES, M. B., *Encounter Groups: First Facts*, Basic Books, New York, 1973.

RAPOPORT, R., *Community as Doctor*, Tavistock, London, 1960.

RICE, A. K., *Learning for Leadership*, Tavistock, London, 1965.

ROGERS, C., *Encounter Groups*, Penguin, Harmondsworth, 1969.

SKYNNER, A. C. R., *One Flesh, Separate Persons*, Constable, London, 1976.

WHITAKER, D. S. and LIEBERMAN, M. A., *Psychotherapy Through the Group Process*, Tavistock, London, 1965.

YALOM, I. D., *The Theory and Practice of Group Psychotherapy*, Basic Books, New York and London, 1970.

Bibliographical index

ABROMS, G. M. (1969). Defining milieu therapy. *Archives of General Psychiatry*, **21**, 553–60. [105]

AHUMADA, J. L. (1976). On limited-time group psychotherapy. II: Group process. *British Journal of Medical Psychology*, 49, 81–8. [29]

AHUMADA, J. L., ABINSO, D., BAIGUERA, N. and GALLO, A. (1974). On limited-time psychotherapy. I: Setting, admission and therapeutic ideology. *Psychiatry*, **37**, 254–80. [29]

ALLPORT, F. H. (1920). The influence of the group upon association and thought. *Journal of Experimental Psychology*, **3**, 159–82. [6]

ALLPORT, F. H. (1924). *Social Psychology*. Houghton Mifflin, Boston. [5] [6]

ALLPORT, F. H. (1934). The J-curve hypothesis of conforming behaviour. *Journal of Social Psychology*, **5**, 141–83. [6]

ARNOLD, WILLIAM R. and STILES, BILL (1972). A summary of increasing use of 'group methods' in correctional institutions. *International Journal of Group Psychothèrapy*. **22** (1), 77–92. [177]

ASCH, S. E. (1951). Effects of group pressure upon the modification and distortion of judgements. In Cartwright and Zander (1960), pp. 189–200. [52]

ASCH, S. E. (1952). *Social Psychology*. Prentice-Hall, Englewood Cliffs, NJ. [52]

ASTRACHAN, B. M. (1970). Towards a social systems model of therapeutic groups, *Social Psychiatry*, **5**, 110–19. [44]

BACH, G. R. (1954). *Intensive group Psychotherapy*. Ronald Press, New York. [80, 81]

BACK, K. (1951). Influence through social communication. *Journal of Abnormal and Social Psychology*, **46**, 9–23. [65]

BALES, R. F. (1950a). *Interaction Process Analysis: A Method for the Study of Small Groups*. Addison Wesley Press, Cambridge, Massachusetts. Partly reprinted as A theoretical framework for interaction process analysis in Cartwright and Zander (1953). [71, 72]

BALES, R. F. (1950b). A set of categories for the analysis of small group interaction. *American Sociological Review*, **15**, 257–63. [71, 73]

BALES, R. F. (1953). The equilibrium problem in small groups. In Parsons,

T., Bales, R. F. and Shils, E. A. *Working Papers in the Theory of Action*. Free Press, New York. Reprinted in Hare *et al*. (1955). [72]

BALES, R. F. (1970). *Personality and Interpersonal Behavior*. Holt, Rinehart and Winston, New York. [71, 73]

BALES, R. F. and SLATER, P. E. (1955). Role differentiation in small decision-making groups. In Parsons, T., Bales, R. F. *et al*., *The Family Socialisation and Interaction Process*. Free Press, New York. [74]

BALES, R. F. and STRODTBECK, F. L. (1951). *Phases in group problem-solving*. *Journal of Abnormal and Social Psychology*, **46**, 485–95. Reprinted in Cartwright and Zander (1968), pp. 389–98. [70, 75]

BALES, R. F., STRODTBECK, F. L., MILLS, T. M. and ROSEBOROUGH, M. E. (1951). Channels of communication in small groups. *American Sociological Review*, **16**, 461–8. [74]

BANNISTER, D. and FRANSELLA, F. (1971). *Inquiring Man: The Theory of Personal Constructs*. Penguin, Harmondsworth. [203, 204]

BANNISTER, D. and MAIR, J. M. M. (1968). *The Evaluation of Personal Constructs*. Academic Press, London. [203, 204]

BARLOW, D. H. and HERSEN, M. (1973). Single-case experimental designs: uses in applied clinical research. *Archives of General Psychiatry*, **29**, 319–25. [191]

BARTON, R. W. A. C. (1959). *Institutional Neurosis*. John Wright, Bristol. [88] [92]

BATESON, GREGORY, JACKSON, DON, MALEY, JOY, WEAKLAND, JOHN (1956). Toward a theory of schizophrenia. *Behavioral Science*, **1**, 251–304. [182]

BAVELAS, A. (1950). Communication patterns in task-oriented groups. *Journal of the Acoustical Society of America*, **22**, 725–30. Reprinted in Cartwright and Zander (1968), pp. 503–11. [43, 70]

BECKETT, J. A. (1973). General systems theory, psychiatry and psychotherapy. *International Journal of Group Psychotherapy*, **23**, 292–305. [43, 44]

BEDNAR, R. L. and LAWLIS, G. F. (1971). Empirical research in group psychotherapy. In Bergin and Garfield, pp. 812–38. [61, 198], 199

BEELS, C. CHRISTIAN and FERBER, ANDREW (1969). Family therapy: a view. *Family Process*, **8** (1), 280–318. [182] 183,

BELKNAP, I. (1956). *Human Problems of a State Mental Hospital*. McGraw-Hill, New York. [88, 92]

BELL, J. (1961). *Family group therapy*, Public Health Monologue, 64. US Department of Health, Education and Welfare, Washington, DC. [183]

BENNIS, W. G. and SHEPARD, H. A. (1956). A theory of group development. *Human Relations*, **9**, 415–37. Reprinted in Gibbard, *et al*. (1974), pp. 127–53. [77]

BERGIN, A. E. (1963). The effects of psychotherapy: negative results revisited. *Journal of Counseling Psychology*, **10**, 244–50. [193]

BERGIN, A. E. (1966). Some implications of psychotherapy research for therapeutic practice. *Journal of Abnormal Psychology*, **71**, 235–46. [193]

BERGIN, A. E. (1967a). An empirical analysis of therapeutic issues. In Arbuckle, D. (ed.) *Counseling and Psychotherapy: An Overview*. McGraw Hill, New York. [193]

BERGIN, A. E. (1967b). Further comments on psychotherapy research and therapeutic practice. *International Journal of Psychiatry*, **3**, 317–23. [193]

BERGIN, A. E. (1970). The deterioration effect: a reply to Braucht. *Journal of Abnormal Psychology*, **75**, 300–02. [193]

BERGIN, A. E. (1971). The evaluation of therapeutic outcomes. In Bergin and Garfield (1971), pp. 217–70. [188], 189, 191, 192, 193, 194, 201

BERGIN, A. E. and GARFIELD, S. L. (eds.) (1971). *Handbook of Psychotherapy and Behavior Change*. John Wiley, New York. [189]

BERGIN, A. E. and SUINN, R. H. (1975). Individual psychotherapy and behaviour therapy. *Annual Review of Psychology*, **26**, 509–56. [201]

BERNARD, L. L. (1924). *Instinct: A Study in Social Psychology*. Holt, Rinehart & Winston, New York. [6]

BERNE, E. (1966). *Principles of Group Treatment*. Oxford University Press, London and New York. [160]

BEUKENKAMP, C. (1952). Some observations made during group therapy. *Psychiatric Quarterly Supplement*, **26**, 22–6. [81]

BION, W. R. (1955). Group dynamics: a review. In Klein, M., Heimann, P. and Money-Kyrle, R. E. (eds.), *New Directions in Psycho-Analysis*, Tavistock, London. [15]

BION, W. R. (1961). *Experiences in Groups*. Tavistock, London. [15, 41], 80, [107], 133

BLAKE, R. R. (1953). The interaction-feeling hypothesis applied to psychotherapy groups. *Sociometry*, **16**, 253–65. [76]

BOCKOVEN, J. S. (1963). *Moral Treatment in American Psychiatry*. Springer, New York. [93]

BORGATTA, E. F. and BALES, R. F. (1956). Sociometric status patterns and characteristics of interaction. *Journal of Social Psychology*, **43**, 289–97. [49]

BOTT, E. (1976). Hospital and society. *British Journal of Medical Psychology*, **49**, 97–140. [89, 90]

BOURNIQUE, G. and BOURNIQUE, J. (1975). Thoughts on the IIIrd European Symposium. *Group Analysis*, **8** (2), 97–8. [140]

BOVILL, DIANA (1972). A trial of group psychotherapy for neurotics. *British Journal of Psychiatry*, **120**, 285–92. [202], 203

BOWEN, MURRAY (1966). The use of family theory in clinical practice. *Comprehensive Psychiatry*, **7**, 345–74. [181]

BOYESEN, G. (1970). Experiences with dynamic relaxation energy and character. *Journal of Bioenergetic Research*, **1** (1), 32. [153]

BRIGGS, DENNIE L. (1972). A transitional therapeutic community for young violent offenders. *Journal of the Howard League*, **13** (3), 171–83. [178]

BUCKLEY, W. (1967). *Sociology and Modern Systems Theory*. Prentice-Hall, Englewood Cliffs, NJ. [45]

BUCKLEY, W. (ed.) (1968). *Modern Systems Research for the Behavioral Scientist*. Aldine, Chicago. [45]

BURCHARD, E., MICHAELS, J. J. and KOTKOV, B. (1948). Criteria for the evaluation of group therapy. *Psychosomatic Medicine*, **10**, 257–74. [194]

BURGES, R. L. (1969). Communication networks and behavioural consequences. *Human Relations*, **22**, 137–59. [70, 71]

BURNHAM, D. L. (1966). The special problem patient: victim or agent of splitting ? *Psychiatry*, **29**, 105–22. [93]

BURROW, T. (1926a). Our mass neurosis. *Psychology Bulletin*, **23**, 305–12. [5]

BURROW, T. (1926b). Insanity a social problem. *American Journal of Sociology*, **32**, 80–7. [14]

BYNG-HALL, JOHN (1973). Family myths used as a defence in conjoint family therapy. *British Journal of Medical Psychology*, **46**, 239–49. [184]

CABRAL, R. and PATON, A. (1975). Evaluation of group therapy: Correlation between clients' and observers' assessments. *British Journal of Psychiatry*, **126**, 475–7. [202]

CAINE, T. M. and SMAIL, D. J. (1966). Attitudes to treatment of medical staff in therapeutic communities. *British Journal of Medical Psychology*, **39**, 329–34. [127]

CAINE, T. M. and SMAIL, D. J. (1969). *The Treatment of Mental Illness*. University of London Press. [111, 124], 204

CAINE, T. M. and WIJESINGHE, B. (1976). Personality, expectancies and group psychotherapy. *British Journal of Psychiatry*, **129**, 384–7. [202], 204

CAMPBELL, J. P. and DUNNETTE, M. D. (1968). Effectiveness of T-group experiences in managerial training and development. *Psychology Bulletin*, **70**, 73–104. [146]

CARTWRIGHT, D. A. (ed.). (1959). *Studies in Social Power*. Institute for Social Research, Ann Arbor, Michigan. [65]

CARTWRIGHT, D. A. (1965). Influence, leadership, control. In March, J. G. (ed.), *Handbook of Organisations*. Rand McNally, Chicago. [65]

CARTWRIGHT, D. A. (1968). The nature of group cohesiveness. In Cartwright and Zander (1968), pp. 91–109. [65]

CARTWRIGHT, D. A. and ZANDER, A. (eds.) (1953). *Group Dynamics Research and Theory*. Row, Peterson, Evanston, Ill. [56, 64]

CARTWRIGHT, D. A. and ZANDER, A. (eds) (1960). *Group Dynamics Research and Theory*, 2nd ed., Tavistock, London. [56, 64]

CARTWRIGHT, D. A. and ZANDER, A. (eds) (1968). *Group Dynamics Research and Theory*, 3rd ed., Tavistock, London. [42, 56, 60, 64, 65, 66, 67]

CARTWRIGHT, D. S. (1956). Note on 'Changes in psychoneurotic patients with and without psychotherapy'. *Journal of Consulting Psychology*, **20**, 403–04. [193]

CAUDILL, W. A. (1958). *The Psychiatric Hospital as a Small Society*, Harvard University Press. [88] [90] [92] [110]

CHAPPLE, E. D. (1942). The measurement of interpersonal behavior. *Transactions of the New York Academy of Science*, **4**, 223–33. [71]

CHAPPELL, M. H. *et al*. (1937). The value of group psychological procedures in the treatment of peptic ulcers. *American Journal of Digestive Diseases and Nutrition*, **3**, 813–17. [13]

CHASSAN, J. B. (1967). *Research Design in Clinical Psychology and Psychiatry*. Appleton-Century-Crofts, New York. [191]

CLARK, A. W. (1967). Patient participation and improvement in a therapeutic community. *Human Relations*, **20** (3), 259–71. [124]

CLARK, A. W. and YEOMANS, N. T. (1969). *Frazer House: Theory, Practice and Evaluation of a therapeutic community*. Springer, New York. [114] [122]

CLARK, D. H. (1965). The therapeutic community: concept, practice and future, *British Journal of Psychiatry*, **3**, (479), 947–54. [111]

CLARKE, R. V. G. and CORNISH, D. B. (1972). *The Controlled Trial in Institutional Research—Paradigm or Pitfall for Penal Evaluations*. Home Office Research Study. 15, HMSO, London. [122]

COCH, L. and FRENCH JR, J. R. P. (1948). Overcoming resistance to change. *Human Relations*, **11**, 512–32. Reprinted in Cartwright and Zander (1968). [66]

COHLER, J. and SHAPIRO, L. (1964). Avoidance patterns in staff–patient interaction on a chronic schizophrenic ward. *Psychiatry*, **27**, 377–88. [92]

COLEMAN, A. (1971). *The Planned Environment in Psychiatric Treatment: a Manual for Ward Design*. Charles Thomas, Springfield, Ill. 125]

COOLEY, C. H. (1909). *Social Organisation. A Study of the Larger Mind*. Scribner, New York. [41]

COOPER, C. L. (1975). How psychologically dangerous are T-groups and encounter groups. *Human Relations*, **28** (3), 249–60. [169]

COPAS, J. B. and WHITELEY, J. S. (1976). Predicting success in the treatment of psychopaths. *British Journal of Psychiatry*, **129**, 388–92. [120] [122] [123]

CORNISH, D. B. and CLARKE, R. V. G. (1975). *Residential Treatment and its Effect on Delinquency*. Home Office Research Study 32, HMSO, London. [122] [124]

CORSINI, R. J. (1957). *Methods of Group Psychotherapy*. McGraw Hill, New York. [80, 81]

CORSINI, R. J. (1966). *Role-playing in Psychotherapy*. Aldine, Chicago. [156]

214

CORTÉS, F., PRZEWORSKI, A. and SPRAGUE, J. (1974). *Systems Analysis for Social Scientists*. John Wiley, New York. [45]

COX, M. (1973). The group therapy interaction chronogram. *British Journal of Social Work*, 3 (2), 243–56. [37]

CRAFT, M., STEPHENSON, G. and GRANGER, O. (1964). A controlled trial of authoritarian and self-governing regimes with adolescent psychopaths. *American Journal of Orthopsychiatry*, 34 (3), 543–54. [122], 180

CROCKET, R. W. (1960). Doctor, administrator and the therapeutic community. *Lancet*, 2, 359–63. [109]

CROCKET, R. W. (1962). Initiation of the therapeutic community approach to treatment in a neurosis centre. *International Journal of Group Psychotherapy*, 12, 180. [109]

CUMMING, J. and CUMMING, E. (1964). *Ego and Milieu*. Tavistock, London. [88, 90, 100], 102

CURRY, A. E. (1967). Large therapeutic groups. *International Journal of Group Psychotherapy*, 17, 536–47. [131]

DEANE, ROSEMARY (1972). Group work in prisons. *Journal of the Howard League*, 13 (3), 246–8. [179]

DE MARÉ, P. B. (1972). Large group psychotherapy: a suggested technique. *Group Analysis* 5 (2), 106–08. [128]

DENTLER, R. A. and ERIKSON, K. T. (1959). The function of deviance in groups. *Social Problems*. 7, 98–107. [52]

DEUTSCH, K. W. (1963). *The Nerves of Government*. Free Press, New York. [47]

DEUTSCH, M. (1949). The effects of co-operation and competition upon group process. *Human Relations*, 2, 129–52 and 199–231. Condensed in Cartwright and Zander (1968), pp. 461–82. [43, 54, 67]

DEUTSCH, M. (1968a). Field theory. In Sills, D. A. (ed.), *International Encyclopedia of the Social Sciences*, Vol. 5. Macmillan and Free Press, New York. [56]

DEUTSCH, M. (1968b). Field theory in social psychology. In Lindzey, G. and Aronson, E. (eds), *The Handbook of Social Psychology*, Vol. 1. Addison-Wesley, Mass. [56]

DEUTSCH, M. and GERARD, H. B. (1955). A study of normative and informational social influences upon individual judgement. *Journal of Abnormal and Social Psychology*, 51, 629–36. Reprinted in Cartwright and Zander (1960), pp. 201–13. [52]

DICK, B. M. (1975). A ten-year study of out-patient analytic group therapy. *British Journal of Psychiatry*, 127, 365–75. [203]

DICKENS, C. (1842). *American Notes for General Circulation*. Chapman and Hall, London. [85]

DICKENS, M. and SOLOMON, R. S. (1938). The J-curve hypothesis: certain aspects clarified. *Sociometry*, 1, 277–91. [6]

DUDYCHA, G. J. (1937). An examination of the J-curve hypothesis based on punctuality distributions. *Sociometry*, 1, 144–54. [6]

DUNPHY, D. C. (1968). Phases, role and myths in self-analytic groups. *Journal of Applied Behavioural Science*, **4**, 195–225. Reprinted in Gibbard, *et al.* (1974). [76]

DURKHEIM, E. (1933). *The Division of Labour in Society* (trans. G. Simpson, 1964), Free Press, New York; Collier Macmillan, London. [41]

DURKHEIM, E. (1952). *Suicide. A Study in Sociology* (trans. J. A. Spaulding and G. Simpson). [41]

DURKIN, H. E. (1957). Toward a common basis for group dynamics: group and therapeutic processes in group psychotherapy, *International Journal of Group Psychotherapy*, **7**, 115–30. [199]

DURKIN, H. E. (1964). *The Group in Depth*. International Universities Press, New York. [57, 72]

DURKIN, H. E. (1972). General systems theory and group therapy: an introduction. *International Journal of Group Psychotherapy*, **22**, 159–66. [44]

EDELSON, M. (1970). *Sociotherapy and Psychotherapy*. University of Chicago Press. [96, 113, 130, 134]

ERIKSON, E. (1950). *Childhood and Society*. Norton, New York. [90]

ETZIONI, A. (1964). *Modern Organisations*. Prentice-Hall, Englewood Cliffs, NJ. [7]

EYSENCK, H. J. (1952). The effects of psychotherapy: an evaluation. *Journal of Consulting Psychology*, **16**, 319–24. [188]

EYSENCK, H. J. (ed.) (1960). *Handbook of Abnormal Psychology*. Pitman, London. [188]

EYSENCK, H. J. (1965). The effects of psychotherapy. *International Journal of Psychiatry*, **1**, 99–144. [188]

EZRIEL, H. (1950). A psychoanalytic approach to group treatment. *British Journal of Medical Psychology*, **23**, 59–74. [17]

EZRIEL, H. (1959). The role of transference in psychoanalytic and other approaches to group treatment. *Acta Psychotherapeutica*, **7**, Suppl. [733]

EZRIEL, H. (1967). The first session in psycho-analytic group treatment. *Nederlands Tijdschrift Voor Geneeskunde*, **III** (15), 711–16. [17]

FAIRWEATHER, G. (ed.) (1964). *Social Psychology in Treating Mental Illness: An Experimental Approach*. John Wiley, New York. [125]

FELDMAN, R. A. (1969). Group integration and intense interpersonal disliking. *Human Relations*, **22**, 405–13. [52]

FERREIRA, A. J. (1963). Family myth and homeostasis. *Archives of General Psychiatry*, **9** (45), 457–63. [185]

FESTINGER, L. (1950). Informal social communication. *Psychological Review*, **57**, 271–82. Reprinted in Cartwright and Zander (1968), pp. 182–91. [52, 65]

FESTINGER, L., SCHACHTER, S. and BACK, K. (1950). *Social Pressures in Informal Groups*. Harper and Row, New York. Partly condensed as

Operation of group standards in Cartwright and Zander (1968), pp. 152-4. [42, 52, 64, 65, 67]

FIEDLER, F. E. (1968). Personality and situational determinants of leadership effectiveness. In Cartwright and Zander (1968), pp. 362-80. [68]

FISHER, SETHARD (1968). Therapeutic community in a correctional establishment. *British Journal of Criminology*, **8** (3), 275-84. [178]

FOULKES, S. H. (1975). *Group Analytic Psychotherapy. Method and Principles*. Gordon & Breach, London. [20]

FOULKES, S. H. and ANTHONY, E. J. (1957). *Group Psychotherapy: The Psycho-analytic Approach*. Penguin, Harmondsworth. [18] [107] [108]

FRANK, J. D. (1957). Some determinants, manifestations and effects of cohesiveness in therapy groups. *International Journal of Group Psychotherapy*, **7**, 53-63. [199]

FRANK, J. D. (1961). *Persuasion and Healing*. John Hopkins Press, Baltimore. [189, 202]

FRANK, J. D. (1968). Recent American research in psychotherapy. *British Journal of Medical Psychology*, **41**, 5-13. [202]

FRANK, J. D. (1975). Group psychotherapy research 25 years later. *International Journal of Group Psychotherapy*, **25**, 159-62. [195]

FRANSELLA, F. (1970). . . . . And then there was one. In Bannister, D. (ed.), *Perspectives in Personal Construct Theory*. Academic Press, London. [204]

FRANSELLA, F. and JOYSTON-BECHAL, M. P. (1971). An investigation of conceptual process and pattern change in a psychotherapy group. *British Journal of Psychiatry*, **119**, 199-206. [204]

FREEMAN, T. (1967). Psychoanalytic psychotherapy in the National Health Service. *British Journal of Psychiatry*, **113**, 321-7. [206]

FRENCH, JR J. R. P. and RAVEN, B. (1959). The bases of social power. In Cartwright (1959). Reprinted in Cartwright and Zander (1968), pp. 259-69. [65]

FREUD, S. (1921). *Group Psychology and the Analysis of the Ego*. (trans. and ed. J. Strachey, 1967). The Hogarth Press and the Institute of Psycho-Analysis, London. [2, 3, 6,] 129, 50

FUREDI, J., SZEGEDI, M., and KUN, M. (1974). Methodological problems of the therapeutic community's large groups. *International Journal of Group Psychotherapy*, **24** (2), 190-8. [130]

GARFIELD, S. L. (1971). Research on client variables in psychotherapy. In Bergin and Garfield, pp. 271-98. [202]

GIBBARD, G. S., HARTMAN, J. J. and MANN, R. D. (eds) (1974). *Analysis of Groups: Contributions to Theory, Research, and Practice*. Jossey Bass, San Francisco and London. [23, 71, 72, 77]

GIBBS, J. R. (1970). The effects of human relations training. In Bergin, A. E. and Garfield, S. L. (eds), *Handbook of Psychotherapy and Behavior Change*, John Wiley, New York. [169]

217

GLATT, MAX M. (1974). Alcoholism: a discussion of some controversial issues. *British Journal of Hospital Medicine*, **11** (1), 111–22. [176]

GOFFMAN, E. (1968). *Asylums. Essays on the Social Situation of Mental Patients and Other Inmates.* Penguin, Harmondsworth. [88, 89, 90, 91, 92, 93, 95, 96, 115]

GOLDSTEIN, A. P. (1962). *Therapist–Patient Expectancies in Psychotherapy.* Pergammon, London. [202]

GOLDSTEIN, A. P. (1966). Psychotherapy research by extrapolation from social psychology. *Journal of Counseling Psychology*, **13**, 38–45. [199]

GOLDSTEIN, A. P., HELLER, K. and SECHREST, L. B. (1966). *Psychotherapy and the Psychology of Behavior Change.* John Wiley, New York. [202]

GOLDSTEIN, A. P. and SIMONSON, N. R. (1971). Social psychological approaches to psychotherapy research. In Bergin and Garfield, pp. 154–95. [199]

GORDON, J. (1976). Unpublished data, Henderson Hospital. [205]

GOTTSCHALK, C. A. (1960). Psychoanalytic notes on T-groups at the Human Relations Laboratory, Bethel, Maine. *Comprehensive Psychiatry*, **71**, 472–87. [169]

GRAY, WILLIAM J. (1974). Grendon Prison. *British Journal of Hospital Medicine*, **12** (3), 299–308. [178]

GREENBLATT, M. (1960). The transitional hospital: a clinical and administrative viewpoint. *Journal of Social Issues*, **16**, 62–9. [88]

GREENBLATT, M., YORK, R. M. and BROWN, E. L. (1955). *From Custodial to Therapeutic Patient Care in Mental Hospitals.* Russell Sage, New York. [88]

GREENE, J. S. (1932). *I was a Stutterer: Stories from Life.* Grafton Press, New York. [13]

GRINKER, R. R. (1969). Preface. In Gray, W., Duhl, F. J. and Rizzo, N. D. (eds), *General Systems Theory and Psychiatry.* Little Brown, Boston. [44]

GROB, G. (1966). *The State and the Mentally Ill: A History of Worcester State Hospital in Massachussetts*, 1830–1920. University of North Carolina Press. [85]

GROTJAHN, M. (1950). The process of maturation in group psychotherapy and in the group therapist. *Psychiatry*, **13**, 63–7. [80, 81]

GUETZKOW, H. (1968). Differentiation of roles in task-orientated groups. In Cartwright and Zander (1968), pp. 512–25. [54]

GUNDLACH, R. H. (1967). Overview of outcome studies in group psychotherapy. *International Journal of Group Psychotherapy*, **17**, 196–210. [198]

HADLEY, S. W. and STRUPP, H. H. (1976). Contemporary views of negative effects in psychotherapy: an integrated account. *Archives of General Psychiatry*, **33**, 1291–1302. [193]

HALL, J. R. (1973). Structural characteristics of a psychiatric patient community. *Human Relations*, **26**, 787–809. [101, 104]

HAND, I., LAMONTAGNE, Y. and MARKS, I. M. (1974). Group exposure (flooding) in vivo for agoraphobics, *British Journal of Psychiatry*, **124**, 588–602. [173]

HARE, A. P. (1962). *Handbook of Small Group Research*. Free Press, New York. [42, 54, 69, 70, 129]

HARE, A. P., BORGATTA, E. F. and BALES, R. F. (eds) (1955). *Small Groups: Studies in Social Interaction*. Knopf, New York. [42, 74, 75]

HARMS, E. (1957). Modern psychotherapy—150 years ago. *Journal of Mental Science*, **103** (433), p. 804–09. [86]

HARRINGTON, J. A. (1970). Much ado about milieu. *Laval Medical*, **41**, 814–20. [105]

HARRIS, T. A. (1973). *I'm O.K. You're O.K.* Pan Books, London. [159, 160]

HARVEY, O. L. (1935). The institutionalisation of human sexual behaviour: a study of frequency distributions. *Journal of Abnormal and Social Psychology*, **29**, 427–33. [6]

HASTINGS, PHILIP and RUNKLE, ROBERT L. (1963). An experimental group of married couples with severe problems. *International Journal of Group Psychotherapy*, **13** (1), 84–92. [186]

HEINICKE, C. and BALES, R. F. (1955). Developmental trends in the structure of small groups. *Sociometry*, **16**, 7–38. [75]

HELLER, K. (1971). Laboratory interview research as an analogue to treatment. In Bergin and Garfield, pp. 126–53. [191]

HENRY, J. (1954). The formal social structure of a psychiatric hospital. *Psychiatry*, **17** (2), 139–51. [88, 91, 93]

HIGGINS, G. (1972). The Scandinavians rehearse the liberation. *Journal of Applied Behavioral Science*, **8**, 6. [148]

HILL, W. F. (ed.) (1961). *Collected Papers on Group Psychotherapy*. Utah State Hospital, Provo, Utah. [76]

HOCH, P. H. and ZUBIN, J. (1964). *The Evaluation of Psychiatric Treatment*. Grune and Stratton, New York. [196]

HODGKIN, NANCY (1972). The new careers project at Vacaville. *Journal of the Howard League*, **13** (3), 184–211. [178]

HOERL, R. T. (1974). Encounter groups: their effect on rigidity. *Human Relations*, **27** (5), 431–8. [169]

HOMANS, G. C. (1951). *The Human Group*, Harcourt Brace, New York, Routledge & Kegan Paul, London. [68]

HOMANS, G. C. (1961). *Social Behaviour: Its Elementary Forms*. Routledge & Kegan Paul, London. [68]

HOMANS, G. H. (1968). Groups: the study of groups. In Sills, D. L. (ed.), *International Encyclopedia of the Social Sciences*, Vol. 6. Macmillan and Free Press, New York. [68]

HOME OFFICE (1966). *Studies in the Course of Delinquency and the Treatment of Offenders: (No. 9) A Survey of Group Work in the Probation Service*. HMSO, London. [180]

HULL, C. L. (1933). *Hypnosis and Suggestibility*. Appleton-Century, New York. [6]

HUNT, J. H. (1964). Concerning the impact of group psychotherapy on psychology. *International Journal of Group Psychotherapy*, **14**, 3–31. [6]

HURWITZ, J. I., ZANDER, A. F. and HYMOVITCH, B. (1968). Some effects of power on the relations among group members. In Cartwright and Zander (1968), pp. 291–7. [64]

JACKINS, H. (1965). *The Human Side of Human Beings: The Theory of Re-evaluation Counseling*. Rational Island, Seattle. [156]

JACKSON, DON D. (1957). The question of family homeostasis. *Psychiatric Quarterly Supplement*, **31**, 79–90. [182]

JACKSON, J. M. (1959). Reference group processes in a formal organisation. *Sociometry*, **22**, 303–27. Reprinted in Cartwright and Zander (1960), pp. 120–40. [52, 59, 64]

JACQUES, E. (1955). Social systems as a defence against persecutory and depressive anxiety. In Klein, M., Heimann, P. and Money-Kyrle, R. E. (eds). *New Directions in Psycho-Analysis*. Tavistock, London. [17]

JANOV, A. (1970). *The Primal Scream*. Putman, New York. [152]

JENNESS, A. (1932a). Social influences in the change of opinion. *Journal of Abnormal and Social Psychology*, **27**, 29–34. [6]

JENNESS, A. (1932b). The role of discussion in changing opinion regarding a matter of fact, *Journal of Abnormal and Social Psychology*, **27**, 279–96. [6]

JENNINGS, H. H. (1950). *Leadership and Isolation*, 2nd ed. Longmans Green, New York. [11]

JONES, HOWARD (1973). Approved schools and attitude change. *British Journal of Criminology*, **13** (2), 148–56. [179]

JONES, M. (1953). *The Therapeutic Community: A New Treatment Method in Psychiatry*. Basic Books, New York. [41, 124]

JONES, M. (1956). The concept of the therapeutic community. *American Journal of Psychiatry*, **112** (8), 647–50. [96, 111]

JONES, M. (1962). *Social Psychiatry in the Community, in Hospitals and in Prisons*. Charles C. Thomas, Springfield, Ill. [177]

JONES, M. (1966). Group work in mental hospitals. *British Journal of Psychiatry*, **112**, 1007–11. [101]

JONES, M. and HOLLINGSWORTH, S. (1963a). The ward meeting. *Proceedings of the IIIrd World Congress of Psychiatry*. Canada. [102]

JONES, M. and HOLLINGSWORTH, S. (1963b). Work with large groups in mental hospitals. *Journal of Individual Psychology*, **19**, 61–8. [102, 130]

JUNG, C. G. (1936). Wotan. In *Collected Works*, 10. [4]

JUNG, C. G. (1938). Psychology and religion. In *Collected Works*, 11. [4]

KELLEY, H. (1951). Communication in experimentally created hierarchies. *Human Relations*, **4**, 39–56. In Cartwright and Zander (1960), pp. 781–99. [64]

KELLEY, G. A. (1955). *The Psychology of Personal Constructs*. Norton, New York. [203]

KERNBERG, O. A. (1975). A systems approach to priority setting of interventions in groups. *International Journal of Group Psychotherapy*, **25**, 251-75. [44, 63]

KESEY, K. (1902). *One Flew Over the Cuckoo's Nest*. Methuen & Co., London. [90]

KIESLER, D. J. A grid model for theory and research in the psychotherapies. In Eron, L. D. and Callahan, R. (eds), *The Relationship of Theory to Practice in Psychotherapy*. Aldine, Chicago. [191]

KIESLER, D. J. (1971). Experimental designs in psychotherapy research. In Bergin and Garfield, pp. 36-74. [188], 189, 190, 191

KING, C. H. (1959). Activity group therapy with a schizophrenic boy—follow-up two years later. *International Journal of Group Psychotherapy*, **9**, 184-94. [80, 81]

KISSIN, B., ROSENBLATT, S. and MACHOVER, S. (1967). In Lipton, Martinson and Wilks (eds). *Prognostic Factors in Alcoholism*. Department of Psychiatry, State University of New York (Mime). [177]

KORTEN, D. C. (1962). Situational determinants of leadership structure. *Journal of Conflict Resolution*, **6**, 222-35. Reprinted in Cartwright and Zander (1968), p. 351-61. [68]

KOTIN, J. and SHARAS, M. R. (1967). Intra-staff controversy at a state mental hospital: an analysis of ideological issues. *Psychiatry*, **31** (1), 16-29. [94]

KOTKOV, B. (1956). Research. In Slavson, S. R. (ed.), *The Fields of Group Psychotherapy*. International University Press, New York. [194]

KREEGER, L. (1974). Introduction. In Kreeger, L. (ed.), *The Large Group. Dynamics and Therapy*. Constable, London. [131]

LAZELL, E. W. (1921). The group treatment of *Dementia praecox*. *Psychoanalytic Review*, **8**, 168-79. [13]

LE BON, G. (1895). *Psychologie des Foules*. Alcan, Paris. Trans: *The Crowd: A Study of the Popular Mind*. Benn, London, 1920. [1], 3, 131

LECKWART, J. E. F. (1968). Social distance: an important variable in psychiatric settings. *Psychiatry*, **31**, 352-61. [92]

LENEER-AXELSON, BARBRO (1969). Group therapy among Swedish recidivists. *Journal of the Howard League*, **12** (4), 297-8. [179]

LENNARD, H. and BERNSTEIN, A. (1960). *The Anatomy of Psychotherapy: Systems of Communication and Expectation*. Columbia University Press. [76]

LETEMENDIA, F. J. J., HARRIS, A. and WILLEMS, J. A. (1967). The clinical effects on a population of chronic schizophrenic patients of administrative changes in a hospital. *British Journal of Psychiatry*, **113**, 959-71. [123]

LEWIN, K. (1935). *A Dynamic Theory of Personality* (trans. D. K. Adams and K. E. Zener), McGraw-Hill, New York. [56]

LEWIN, K. (1936). *Principles of Topological Psychology*. McGraw-Hill, New York. [56, 57]

LEWIN, K. (1943). Forces behind food habits and methods of change. *Bulletin of the National Research Council*, **108**, 35–65. See also Studies in group decision. In Cartwright and Zander (1953). [57, 63]

LEWIN, K. (1944). Constructs in psychology and psychological ecology. University of Iowa Studies in Child Welfare, **20** (409), 1–49. [40]

LEWIN, K. (1947a). Group decision and social change. In Newcomb, T. M. and Hartly, E. L. (eds), *Readings in Social Psychology*. Holt, Rinehart & Winston, New York. [57]

LEWIN, K. (1947b). Frontiers in group dynamics: concept, method and reality in social science; social equilibria and social change. *Human Relations*, **1**, 5–41. [58, 62]

LEWIN, K. (1947c). Frontiers in group dynamics II. Channels of group life; social planning and action research. *Human Relations*, **1**, 143–53. [58], 59, 60, 63

LEWIN, K. (1948). *Resolving Social Conflicts: Selected Papers on Group Dynamics*. Harper Brothers, New York. [58]

LEWIN, K. (1951). *Field Theory in Social Science*. Harper Brothers, New York. [19, 57, 58, 129]

LEWIN, K. and LIPPIT, R. (1938). An experimental approach to the study of autocracy and democracy: a preliminary note. *Sociometry*, **1**, 292–300. [60]

LEWIN, K., LIPPITT, R. and WHITE, R. K. (1939). Patterns of aggressive behaviour in experimentally created 'social climate'. *Journal of Social Psychology*, 10, 271–99. [60]

LEWIS, P. and MCCANTS, J. (1973). Some current issues in group psychotherapy research. *International Journal of Group Psychotherapy*, **23**, 282–8. [197]

LIDZ, THEODORE, CORNELISON, A., FLECK, S. and TERRY, D. (1957). The intrafamilial environment of schizophrenic patients. *American Journal of Psychiatry*, **114**, 241–8. [182]

LIEBERMAN, M. A., YALOM, I. D. and MILES, M. B. (1973). *Encounter Groups: First Facts*. Basic Books, New York. [170]

LINDSAY, J. S. B. (1972). On the number in a group. *Human Relations*, **25**, 47–64. [41]

LIPPITT, R. (1939). Field theory and experiment in social psychology: autocratic and democratic group atmosphere. *American Journal of Sociology*, **45**, 26–49. [60]

LIPPIT, R., POLANSKY, N., REDL, F. and ROSEN, S. (1952). The dynamics of power. *Human Relations*, **5**, 37–64. Reprinted in Cartwright and Zander (1968), pp. 236–50. [50]

LIPTON, DOUGLAS, MARTINSON, ROBERT and WILKS, JUDITH (1975). *The Effectiveness of Correctional Treatment*. Praeger. New York, Washington and London. [180, 181]

LISS, J. (1974a). *Free to Feel.* Wildwood House, London. [144]

LISS, J. (1974b). Co-operative help: the art of helpful listening. Unpublished paper. [158]

LOCKE, N. M. (1961). *Group Psychoanalysis.* University Press, New York. [34]

LOEB, M. B. (1956). Some dominant and cultural themes in a psychiatric hospital. *Social Problems,* **4**, 17–20. [95]

LOWEN, A. (1966). *The Betrayal of the Body.* Macmillan, New York. [153]

LUBIN, B., LUBIN, A. W. and SARGENT, C. W. (1972). The group psychotherapy literature, 1971. *International Journal of Group Psychotherapy,* **22**, 492–529. [195]

MCCANCE, C. and MCCANE, P. F. (1969). Alcoholism in north east Scotland: its treatment and outcome. *British Journal of Psychiatry,* **115** (519), 189–98. [176]

MCDOUGALL, W. (1920). *The Group Mind.* Cambridge University Press. [5, 6]

MCCOWEN, P. and WILDER, J. (1975). *Life Style of 100 Psychiatric Patients.* Psychiatric Rehabilitation Centre, London. [103]

MAIN, T. F. (1946). The hospital as a therapeutic institution. *Bulletin of the Meminger Clinic,* **10** (3), 66–70. [41, 88, 92, 96, 107, 109, 110]

MAIN, T. F. (1957). The ailment. *British Journal of Medical Psychology,* **30**, 129–45. [93]

MAIN, T. F. (1974). Some psycho-dynamics of large groups. In Kreeger, L. (ed.), *The Large Group,* Constable, London. [132]

MALAN, D. H. (1959). On assessing the results of psychotherapy. *British Journal of Medical Psychology,* **32**, 86–105. [189]

MALAN, D. H. (1963). *A Study of Brief Psychotherapy.* Tavistock, London. [192]

MALAN, D. H. (1973). The outcome problem in psychotherapy research. *Archives of General Psychiatry,* **29**, 719–29. [188], 189, 192, 193, 195, 208

MALAN, D. H. (1976a). *Toward the Validation of Dynamic Psychotherapy. A Replication.* Plenum, New York. [192]

MALAN, D. H. (1976b). *The Frontier of Brief Psychotherapy. An Example of The Convergence of Research and Clinical Practice.* Plenum, New York. [192]

MALAN, D. H., BACAL, H. A., HEATH, E. S. *et al.* (1968). A study of psychodynamic changes in untreated neurotic patients: 1. Improvements that are questionable on dynamic criteria. *British Journal of Psychiatry,* **114**, 525–51. [192]

MALAN, D. H., BACAL, H. A., HEATH, E. S. *et al.* (1973). A study of psychodynamic changes in untreated neurotic patients: II. Apparently genuine improvements. *Archives of General Psychiatry,* **32**, 111–26. [192]

223

MALAN, D. H., BALFOUR, F. H. G., HOOD, V. G. and SHOOTER, A. M. N. (1976). Group psychotherapy: a long-term follow-up study. *Archives of General Psychiatry*, **33**, 1303–15. [207]

MANN, J. and SEMRAD, E. V. (1948). The use of group therapy in psychoses. *Journal of Social Casework*, **29**, 176–81. [80]

MANN, R. D. (1966). The development of the member–trainer relationship in self-analytic groups. *Human Relations*, **19**, 85–115. [78]

MANN, R. D., GIBBARD, G. S. and HARTMAN, J. J. (1967). *Interpersonal Styles and Group Development*. John Wiley, New York. [78]

MANN, S. (1975). The 'new long stay' in mental hospitals. *British Journal of Hospital Medicine*, **14** (1), 56–64. [97]

MANNING, N. (1976). Values and practice in the therapeutic community. *Human Relations*, **29** (2), 125–38. [117]

MANOR, O. (1977). Social roles and behavioural change. Unpublished thesis, London University and Henderson Hospital. [117]

MARATOS, JASON and KENNEDY, MARGARET J. (1974). Evaluation of ward group meetings in a psychiatric unit of a general hospital. *British Journal of Psychiatry*, **125**, 479–82. [101]

MARCH, J. G. and SIMON, H. A. (1958). *Organisations*. John Wiley, New York. [59]

MARCUS, B. (1969). Correlates of attitudes to group work. *British Journal of Criminology*, **9** (3), 272–81. [179]

MARGOLIS, P. M. (1973). *Patient Power: The Development of a Therapeutic Community in a Psychiatric Unit of a General Hospital*. Charles C. Thomas, Springfield, Ill. [114]

MAROHN, R. C. (1967). The unit meeting. Its implications for a therapeutic correctional community. *International Journal of Group Psychotherapy*, **17** (2), 159–67. [130]

MARSH, L. C. (1931). Group treatment by the psychological equivalent of the revival. *Mental Hygiene*, **15**, 328–49. [13]

MARTIN, D. V. and CAINE, T. M. (1963). Personality change in the treatment of chronic neurosis in a therapeutic community. *British Journal of Psychiatry*, **109** (459), 267–72. [124]

MARTIN, E. A. and HILL, W. F. (1957). Toward a theory of group development. *International Journal of Group Psychotherapy*, 7, 20–30. [76, 80, 81]

MATZA, D. (1969). *Becoming Deviant*. Prentice-Hall, Englewood Cliffs, NJ. [120]

MAYO, E. (1933). *The Human Problems of an Industrial Civilization*. Macmillan, New York. [7]

MAYS, J. B. (1959). *On the Threshold of Delinquency*. Liverpool University Press. [180]

MEAD, G. H. (1934). *Mind, Self and Society: From the Standpoint of a Social Behaviorist*. University of Chicago Press. [6]

MEARES, R. (1973). Two kinds of groups. *British Journal of Medical Psychology*, **46** (4), 373–80. [14]

MELTZOFF, J. and KORNREICH, M. (1970). *Research in Psychotherapy*. Atherton Press, New York. [189, 195, 207]

MENNINGER, W. (1939). Psychoanalytic principles in psychiatric hospital therapy. *Southern Medical Journal*, **32**, 348–54. [106]

MENZIES, I. (1960). A case-study in the functioning of social systems as a defence against anxiety. *Human Relations*, **13**, 95–121. [17]

MILES, A. (1969a). The effects of a therapeutic community on the interpersonal relationships of a group of psychopaths. *British Journal of Criminology*, **9** (1), 22–38. [122]

MILES, A. (1969b). Changes in the attitudes to authority of patients with behaviour disorders in a therapeutic community. *British Journal of Psychiatry*, **115**, 1049–57. [122]

MILES, A. (1972). The development of interpersonal relationships among long stay patients in two hospital workshops. *British Journal of Medical Psychology*, **45** 105–14. [103, 124]

MILLER, J. G. (1955). Toward a general theory for the behavioral sciences. *American Psychological Journal*, **10**, 513–31. [43, 44]

MILLER, J. G. (1957). Mental health implications of a general behavior theory. *American Journal of Psychiatry*, **113**, 776–82. [43, 44]

MILLER, J. G. (1965a). Living systems: basic concepts. *Behavioral Science*, **10**, 193–237. [43, 44]

MILLER, J. G. (1965b). Living systems: structure and process: cross-level hypotheses. *Behavioral Science*, **10**, 337–411. [43, 44]

MILLER, N. E. and DOLLARD, J. (1941). *Social Learning and Imitation*. Yale University Press. [6]

MILLS, T. M. (1953). Power relations in three-person groups. *American Sociological Review*, **18**, 351–7. Reprinted in Cartwright and Zander (1960), pp. 766–80. [41]

MILLS, T. M. (1962). *The Sociology of Small Groups*. Prentice-Hall, Englewood Cliffs, NJ. [5, 46, 47, 48, 51, 52, 53, 55, 56, 59, 63]

MINSKY, M. (1967). *Computation, Finite and Infinite Machines*. Prentice-Hall, Englewood Cliffs, NJ. [44]

MINUCHIN, S., MONTALVO, B., GUERNEY, B., ROSMAN, B. and SHUMER, F. (1967). *Families of the Slums*. Basic Books, New York. [183]

MISHLER, E. and TRAPP, A. (1956). Status and interaction in a psychiatric hospital. *Human Relations*, **9**, 187–205. [93]

MOOS, R. H. (1974). *Evaluating Treatment Environments*. John Wiley, New York. [89, 124, 192]

MORENO, J. L. (1923). *The Theatre of Spontaneity*. (trans. 1947). Beacon House, Beacon, NY. [71]

MORENO, J. L. (1932). *Application of the Group Method of Classification*. National Committee on Prisons and Prison Labour, New York. [14]

MORENO, J. L. (1934). *Who Shall Survive?* Nervous and Mental Diseases Publishing Co., Washington, DC. Revised ed. (1953), Beacon House, Beacon, NY. [11]

MORENO, J. L. (1941). Foundations of sociometry, an introduction. *Sociometry*, **4**, 15–36. [11]

MORENO, J. L. (1946). *Psychodrama*. Beacon House, Beacon, NY. [155]

MORENO, J. L. (1947). Contributions of sociometry to research methodology in sociology. *American Sociological Review*, **12**, 287–92. [11]

MORENO, J. L. (1951). *Sociometry, Experimental Method and the Science of Society*. Beacon House, Beacon, NY. [11]

MORENO, J. L. (1954). Old and new trends in sociometry: turning points in small group research. *Sociometry*, **17**, 179–93. [11]

MORENO, J. L. and JENNINGS, H. H. (1944). Sociometric methods of grouping and re-grouping; with reference to authoritative and democratic method of grouping. *Sociometry*, **7**, 397–414. [11]

MORGAN, R. and CHEADLE, A. J. (1972). Staff vs patients: the phenomenon of rejection. *British Journal of Medical Psychology*, **121**, 627–34. [94]

MORRICE, J. K. (1972). Myth and the democratic process. *British Journal of Medical Psychology*, **45**, 327–31. [118]

MUMBY, T. (1974). Large groups in industry. In Kreeger, L. (ed.), *The Large Group*, Constable, London. [140]

MUNZER, J. and GREENWALD, H. (1957). Interaction process analysis of a therapy group. *International Journal of Group Psychotherapy*, **7**, 175–90. [76]

MURRAY, HENRY A. (1951). Toward a classification of interactions. Parsons and Shils (1951). [49]

MYERS, K. and CLARK, D. H. (1972). Results in a therapeutic community. *British Journal of Psychiatry*, **120**, 51–8. [122, 123]

MYRDAL, G. (1944). *An American Dilemma*, Harper & Row, New York. [41]

NEWCOMB, T. M. (1943). *Personality and Social Change*. Dryden, New York. [9]

NEWCOMB, T. M. (1958). Attitude Development As A Function of Reference Groups. In *Readings in Social Psychology*, E. E. Maccoby, T. M. Newcomb, and E. L. Hartley (eds), Henry Holt & Company, New York. [9]

O'BRIEN, W. J. (1961). *Personality Assessment as a Measure of Change Resulting from Group Psychotherapy with Male Juvenile Delinquents*. Institute for the Study of Crime and Delinquency and the Californian Youth Authority. [180]

PARKER, S. (1958). Leadership patterns in a psychiatric ward. *Human Relations*, **11**, 287–301. [81]

PARLOFF, M. B. (1961). Therapist–patient relationships and outcome of psychotherapy. *Journal of Consulting Psychology*, **25**, 29–38. [196]

PARLOFF, M. B. (1967). A view from the bridge: group process and outcome. *International Journal of Group Psychotherapy*, **17**, 236–42. [195, 196]

PARLOFF, M. B. (1970a). Assessing the effects of headshrinking and mindexpanding. *International Journal of Group Psychotherapy*, **20**, 14–24. [196, 197]

PARLOFF, M. B. (1970b). Group therapy and the small group field: an encounter. *International Journal of Group Psychotherapy*, **20** (3), 267–304. [169, 170]

PARLOFF, M. B. (1973). Some current issues in group psychotherapy research: discussion. *International Journal of Group Psychotherapy*, **23**, 282–8. [197]

PARSONS, T. (1951a). *The Social System*. Free Press, New York; Collier-Macmillan, London. [45]

PARSONS, T. (1951b). Illness and the role of the physician· a sociological perspective. *American Journal of Orthopsychiatry*. **21**, 452–460. [89]

PARSONS, T. (1968). Social systems. In Sills, D. L. (ed.), *International Encyclopedia of the Social Sciences*, vol. 15, Macmillan and Free Press, New York. [45]

PARSONS, T., BALES, R. F. and SHILS, E. A. (1953). *Working Papers in the Theory of Action*. Free Press, Chicago. [88]

PARSONS, T. and SHILS, E. (eds.) (1951). *Toward a General Theory of Action*. Harper & Row, New York, Collier-Macmillan, London. [45, 46]

PATTISON, E. M. (1965). Evaluation studies in group psychotherapy. *International Journal of Group Psychotherapy*, **15**, 382–97. [195], 197, 198

PAUL, G. L. (1967). Strategy of outcome research in psychotherapy. *Journal of Consulting Psychology*, **31**, 109–18. [190]

PAUL, N. (1967). The role of mourning and empathy in conjoint marital therapy. In Zuk, G. and Boszormenyi-Nagy, I. (eds), *Family Therapy and Disturbed Families*, Palo Alto, Science and Behaviour Books. [183]

PEPITONE, A. and REICHLING, G. (1955). Group cohesiveness and the expression of hostility. *Human Relations*, **8**, 327–37. In Cartwright and Zander (1960), pp. 141–61. [65, 67]

PERLS, F., HEFFERLINE, R. F. and GOODMAN, P. (1973). *Gestalt Therapy*. Penguin, Harmondsworth. [144, 153]

PERSONS, ROY W. and PEPINSKY, HAROLD B. (1966). Convergence in psychotherapy with delinquent boys, *Journal of Counseling Psychology*, **13** (3), 329–34. [180]

PHILLIPSON, H. (1958). The assessment of progress after at least two years of group psychotherapy. *British Journal of Medical Psychology*, **31**, 32–42. [206]

PHOENIX HOUSE (1971). *Information for Professionals. Featherstone Lodge Project*. Phoenix House, London. [174]

PIAGET, J. (1926). *The Language and Thought of the Child*. Harcourt Brace, New York. [71]

PINES, M. (1974). Overview. In Kreeger, L. (ed.) *The Large Group*. Constable, London. [131]

PITTMAN, F. S., DE YOONG, C. F., COMENHAFT, K., KAPLAN, D. M. and LANGSLEY, D. G. (1966). Crisis family therapy. *Current Psychiatric Therapies*, **6**, (ed. Masserman, J. H.), 187–96. [185]

POLANSKY, N., LIPPIT, R. and REDL, F. (1950). An investigation of behavioural contagion in groups. *Human Relations*, **3**, 319–48. [50]

POLANSKY, N. A., WHITE, R. B., MILLER, S. C. (1957). Determinants of the role-image of the patient in a psychiatric hospital. In Greenblatt, M., Levinson, D. J. and Williams, R. H. (eds), *The Patient and the Mental Hospital*. Free Press, Glencoe, Ill. [100]

POWDERMAKER, F. and FRANK, J. D. (1948). Group psychotherapy with neurotics. *American Journal of Psychiatry*, **105**, 449–55. [80, 81]

PRATT, J. H. (1907). The class method of treating consumption in the homes of the poor. *Journal of the American Medical Association*, **49**, 755–9. [13]

PSATHAS, G. (1960a). Interaction process analysis of two psychotherapy groups. *International Journal of Group Psychotherapy*, **10**, 430–45. [76]

PSATHAS, G. (1960b). Phase movement and equilibrium tendencies in interaction process in psychotherapy groups. *Sociometry*, **23**, 177–94. [76]

QUERY, W. T. (1964). Self-disclosure as a variable in group psychotherapy. *International Journal of Group Psychotherapy*, **14**, 107–15. [32]

RABIN, H. M. (1970). Preparing patients for group psychotherapy. *International Journal of Group Psychotherapy*, **20** (2), 135–45. [26]

RAPOPORT, A. (1959). Critique of game theory. *Behavioral Science*, **1**, 303–15. [44]

RAPOPORT, A. (1968). Systems theory. In Sills, D. L. (ed.), *International Encyclopedia of the Social Sciences*, Vol. 15. Macmillan and Free Press, New York. [44]

RAPOPORT, R. (1960). *Community as Doctor*. Tavistock, London. [102, 110, 121, 125]

RAPPARD, PH., AYME, J. and TORRUBIA, H. (1964). (eds). *Encyclopedie Francaise de Psychiatrie*, Therapeutique Institutionelle, 37930 G.10. [86, 88]

RATHOD, N., GREGORY, E., BLOWS, D. and THOMAS, G. H. (1966). A two-year follow-up study of alcoholic patients. *British Journal of Psychiatry*, **112** (488), 683–92. [176]

RAVEN, B. H. and RIETSEMA, J. (1957). The effects of varied clarity of group goal and group path upon the individual and his relation to his group. *Human Relations*, **10**, 29–44. Reprinted in Cartwright and Zander (1960), pp. 395–413. [54]

REDDY, W. B. (1970). Sensitivity training or group psychotherapy: the need for adequate screening. *International Journal of Group Psychotherapy*, **20** (3), 366–71. [169, 170]

REDDY, W. B. and LANSKY, L. M. (1974). The group psychotherapy research: 1973. *International Journal of Group Psychotherapy*, **24**, 477–517. [171, 195]

REDDY, W. B., COLSON, D. B. and KEYS, C. B. (1975). The group psychotherapy literature: 1974. *International Journal of Group Psychotherapy*, **25**, 429–79. [195]

REDDY, W. B. (1976). The group psychotherapy literature: 1975. *International Journal of Group Psychotherapy*, **26**, 487–545. [195]

REDL, F. (1942). Group emotion and leadership. *Psychiatry*, **5**, 573–96. [50]

REES, T. P. (1957). Back to moral treatment and community care. *Journal of Mental Science*, **431** (103), 303–13. [84, 86, 87]

REICH, W. (1949). *Character Analysis*. Farrar, Straus and Givoux, New York. [151]

REPORT OF THE ENQUIRY INTO ST AUGUSTINE'S HOSPITAL. (1976). South-East Thames Regional Health Authority. [89]

REPORT OF THE ENQUIRY INTO DARLINGTON MEMORIAL HOSPITAL. (1976). Newcastle and Durham Regional Health Authority. [89]

RICE, A. K. (1951). The use of unrecognised cultural mechanisms in an expanding machine shop. *Human Relations*, **4**, 143–60. [135]

RICE, A. K. (1963). *The Enterprise and Its Environment*. Tavistock, London. [64]

RICE, A. K. (1965). *Learning for Leadership*. Tavistock, London. [64, 147]

RICHARDSON, J. T., MAYHEW, JR B. A., GRAY, L. N. (1969). Differentiation, restraint and the assymetry of power. *Human Relations*, **22**, 263–74. [49]

RIGHTON, P. (1975). Planned environment therapy: a re-appraisal. *Journal of the Association of Workers for Maladjusted Children*. Spring 1975. [106]

RINGWALD, J. W. (1974). An investigation of group reaction to central figures. In Gibbard, Hartman and Mann (1974), pp. 220–46. [50]

RIOCH, M. J. (1970). Group relations: rationale and technique. *International Journal of Group Psychotherapy*, **20** (3), 340–56. [148]

ROBERTS, B. H. and STRODTBECK, F. L. (1953). Interaction process differences between groups of paranoid schizophrenic and depressed patients. *International Journal of Group Psychotherapy*. **3**, 29–41. [76]

ROCKWELL, D. A. (1971). Some observations on 'living-in'. *Psychiatry*, **34**, 214–23. [89, 93]

ROETHLISBERGER, F. J. and DICKSON, W. J. (1939). *Management and the Worker*. Harvard University Press. [7, 42]

ROGERS, C. R. (1957). The necessary and sufficient conditions of therapeutic personality change. *Journal of Consulting Psychology*, **21** (2), 95–103. [150, 204]

ROGERS, C. R. (1973). *Encounter Groups.* Penguin, Harmondsworth. [143, 149, 168]

ROWLAND, J. (1938). Interaction processes in the state mental hospital. *Psychiatry*, **1**, 323–37. [95, 103]

RUBINSTEIN, E. A. and PARLOFF, M. B. (eds) (1959). *Research in Psychotherapy.* American Psychological Association, Washington DC. [189]

RUESCH, J. and PRESTWOOD, A. R. (1950). Interaction processes and personal codification. *Journal of Personality*, **18**, 391–430. [71]

RYLE, A. (1975). *Frames and Cages: The Repertory Grid Approach to Human Understanding.* Sussex University Press. [204]

RYLE, A. and LIPSHITZ, S. (1976). An intensive case-study of a therapeutic group. *British Journal of Psychiatry*, **128**, 581–7. [204]

SANDERS, R., SMITH, R. and WEINMANN, B. (1967). *Chronic Psychoses and Recovery. An Experiment in Socio-environmental Treatment.* Jossey Bass, San Francisco. [125]

SATIR, VIRGINIA (1967). *Conjoint Family Therapy. A Guide to Theory and Technique.* Science and Behaviour Books, Palo Alto, CA. [182, 183]

SCHACHTER, S., ELLERTSON, N., MCBRIDE, D. and GREGORY, D. (1951). An experimental study of cohesiveness and productivity. *Human Relations*, **4**, 229–38. Reprinted in Cartwright and Zander (1968), pp. 192–8. [43, 65]

SCHIFF, S. B. and GLASSMAN, S. M. (1969). Large and small group therapy in a state mental hospital center. *International Journal of Group Psychotherapy*, **19** (2), 150–7. [134]

SCHINDLER, R. (1958). Bifocal group therapy. In Masserman, J. and Moreno, J. E. (eds), *Progress in Psychotherapy*, Vol. 3. Grune & Stratton, New York. [80, 81]

SCHNEIDER, L. A. (1955). A proposed conceptual integration of group dynamics and therapy. *Journal of Social Psychology*, **42**, 173–91. [199]

SCHUTZ, W. C. (1958). *FIRO: a three-dimensional Theory of Interpersonal Behaviour.* Holt, Rinehart & Winston, New York. [77]

SCHUTZ, W. (1971). *Here Comes Everyone.* Harper & Row, New York. [153]

SCHUTZ, W. (1973). *Joy. Expanding Human Awareness.* Pelican, Harmondsworth. [162]

SCHWARTZ, M. S. and SHOCKLEY, E. L. (1956). *The Nurse and the Mental Patient.* Russell Sage Foundation, New York. [93]

SCHWARTZ, M. S. and WILL, G. T. (1953). Low morale and mutual withdrawal on a mental hospital ward. *Psychiatry*, **16**, 337–53. [93]

SECKEL, JOACHIM P. (1965). *Experiments in Group Counseling with Two Youth Authority Institutions.* Research Report No. 46, California Youth Authority. [180]

SETHNA, E. R. and HARRINGTON, J. A. (1971). Evaluation of group psychotherapy. *British Journal of Psychiatry*, **118**, 641–58. [201, 202]

SHANNON, C. E. and WEAVER, W. (1949). *The Mathematical Theory of Communication.* University Press of Illinois. [44]

SHAPIRO, A. K. (1971). Placebo effects in medicine, psychotherapy and psychoanalysis. In Bergin and Garfield (1971), pp. 439–73. [189]

SHAPIRO, D. A. (1976). The effects of therapeuptic conditions: positive results revisited. *British Journal of Medical Psychology*, **49**, 315–23. [201]

SHELDRAKE, R. and TURNER, B. (1963). Perceptions and factions in a therapeutic community. *Human Relations*, **26**, 371–85. [93]

SHELLOW, R. S., WARD, J. L. and RUBENFELD, S. (1958). Group therapy and the institutionalised delinquent. *International Journal of Group Psychotherapy*, **8**, 265–75. [81]

SHERIF, M. (1936). *The Psychology of Social Norms.* (Harper Torchbook edn. 1966), Harper & Row, New York. [7, 8, 52]

SHERIF, M. and SHERIF, C. W. (1953). *Groups in Harmony and Tension.* Harper & Row, New York. [42]

SHERWOOD, M. (1964). Bion's experiences in groups: a critical evaluation. *Human Relations*, **17** (2), 113–30. [17]

SHLIEN, J. M. *et al.* (1968). *Research in Psychotherapy*, Vol. 3. American Psychological Association, Washington, DC. [189]

SIEGEL, A. E. and SIEGEL, S. (1957). Reference groups, membership groups and attitude change. *Journal of Abnormal and Social Psychology*, **55**, 360–4. Reprinted in Cartwright and Zander (1968), pp. 74–9. [42]

SIMMEL, G. (1902). The number of members as determining the sociological form of the group (trans. A. W. Small). *American Journal of Sociology*, **8**, 1–46, 158–96. [41]

SIMMEL, G. (1950). *The Sociology of George Simmel* (ed. K. H. Wolf). Free Press, Glencoe, Ill. [41]

SIMMEL, G. (1955). *Conflict: The Web of Group Affiliations* (trans. K. H. Wolf). Free Press, Glencoe, Ill. [41]

SKYNNER, A. C. R. (1969). A group-analytic approach to conjoint family therapy. *Journal of Child Psychology and Psychiatry*, **10**, 81–126. [184]

SKYNNER, A. C. R. (1971). A large group experience at the 1970/71 course in group work. *Group Analysis*, **4** (3), 174–6. [140]

SKYNNER, A. C. R. (1974). Boundaries. *Social Work Today*, **5** (10), 290–4. [184]

SKYNNER, A. C. R. (1975). Marital problems and their treatment. *Proceedings of the Royal Society of Medicine*, **68** (7), 405–08. [187]

SKYNNER, A. C. R., SKYNNER, P. and HYATT-WILLIAMS, S. (1975). Is there a spouse in the house? *Group Analysis*, **8** (2), 87–92. [186]

SLATER, P. E. (1966). *Microcosm: structural, Psychological and Religious Evolution in Groups.* John Wiley, New York. [78]

SLAVSON, S. R. (1959). The era of group psychotherapy. *Acta Psychotherapeutica*, **7**, 167–96. [14]

SLAVSON, S. R. (1962). A critique of the group therapy literature. *Acta Psychotherapeutica*, **10**, 62–73. [194]

SMAIL, D. J. (1972). A grid measure of empathy in a therapeutic group. *British Journal of Medical Psychology*, **45**, 165–9. [204]

SMALL, N. (1974). Dependence on opiates. MSW Dissertation, University of Sussex. [174, 175]

SPRINGMANN, R. (1970). A large group. *International Journal of Group Psychotherapy*, **20** (2), 210–18. [131]

SPRINGMANN, R. (1974). Psychotherapy in the large group. In Kreeger, L. (ed.), *The Large Group*. Constable, London. [133, 139]

STANNARD, D. L. (1973). Ideological conflict on a psychiatric ward. *Psychiatry*, **36** (2), 143–56. [89]

STANTON, A. H. and SCHWARTZ, M. S. (1954). *The Mental Hospital*. Basic Books, New York. [88, 90, 91, 93, 94, 110, 131]

STATISTICAL AND RESEARCH REPORT NO. 12 (1973). *Psychiatric Hospitals and Units in England*. HMSO, London. [97]

STEIN, J. W. (1969). *The Family as a Unit of Study and Treatment*. Regional Rehabilitation Research Institute, University of Washington Press. [181]

STOCK, D. and THELEN, H. A. (1958). *Emotional Dynamics and Group Culture*. National Training Publications, Washington. [76]

STOTLAND, E. and KOBLER, A. L. (1965). *Life and Death of a Mental Hospital*. University of Washington Press. [95]

STRODTBECK, F. L. and HARE, A. P. (1954). Bibliography of small group research: from 1900 through 1953. *Sociometry*, **17**, 107–78. [42]

STRUPP, H. H. (1973). The experiential group and the psychotherapeutic enterprise. *International Journal of Group Psychotherapy*, **23**, 115–24. [171]

STRUPP, H. H. and BERGIN, A. E. (1969). Some empirical and conceptual bases for co-ordinated research in psychotherapy: a critical review of issues, trends and evidence. *International Journal of Psychiatry*, **7**, 18–90. [189]

STRUPP, H. H. and LUBORSKY, L. (eds) (1962). *Research in Psychotherapy*, Vol. 2. American Psychological Association, Washington, DC. [189]

SULLIVAN, H. S. (1931). Socio-psychiatric research: its implication for the schizophrenia problem and mental hygiene. *American Journal of Psychiatry*, **10**, 977–91. [106]

SYZ, H. (1961). A summary note on the work of Trigant Burrow. *International Journal of Social Psychiatry*, **7** (4), 292–8. [14]

TALBOT, E. and MILLER, S. C. (1966). The struggle to create a sane society in the psychiatric hospital. *Psychiatry*, **29**, 165–71. [89]

TALBOT, E., MILLER, S. C. and WHITE, R. B. (1964). Some antitherapeutic side effects of hospitalisation and psychotherapy. *Psychiatry*, **27**, 170–6. [95, 96]

TALLAND, G. A. (1955). Task and interaction process: some characteristics of therapeutic group discussion. *Journal of Abnormal and Social Psychology*, **50**, 105–09. Reprinted in Hare, *et al.* (1955). [75]

TAYLOR, A. J. W. (1967). An evaluation of group psychotherapy in a girls' Borstal. *International Journal of Group Psychotherapy*, **17** (2), 168–77. [180]

TEICHER, A., DE FREITAS, L. and OSHERSON, A. (1974). Group psychotherapy and the intense group experience. a preliminary rationale for encounter as a therapeutic agent in the mental health field. *International Journal of Group Psychotherapy*, **35** (2), 159–73. [170]

THELEN, H. A. (1954). *Dynamics of Groups at Work*. University of Chicago Press. [76]

THELEN, H. A. *et al.* (1954). *Methods for Studying Work and Emotionality in Group Operation*. Human Dynamics Laboratory, Chicago. [76]

THOMAS, E. J. (1957). Effects of facilitative role interdependence on group functioning. *Human Relations*, **10**, 347–66. Reprinted in Cartwright and Zander (1960), pp. 347–66. [43, 54, 67]

THOMAS, W. I. and ZNANIECKI, F. (1918). *The Polish Peasant in Europe and America*, Vols. 1–4. University of Chicago Press. [41]

THOMPSON, J. D. and MCEWEN, W. J. (1958). Organisational goals and environment: goal settings as an interaction process. *American Sociological Review*, **23**, 23–31. Reprinted in Cartwright and Zander (1960), pp. 472–84. [53]

THRASHER, F. (1927). *The Gang*. University of Chicago Press. [41]

THRASHER, J. H. and SMITH, H. L. (1964). Interactional contexts of psychiatric patients: social roles and organisational implications. *Psychiatry*, **27**, 389–98. [99]

TOLLINTON, H. J. (1969). The organisation of a psychotherapeutic community. *British Journal of Medical Psychology*, **42**, 271–5. [109]

TOSQUELLES, F. (1964). In Rappard *et al.*, 37930; G10. [97]

TRUAX, C. B. and CARCKHUFF, R. F. (1967). *Toward Effective Counseling and Psychotherapy*. Aldine, Chicago. [189, 200, 201, 204]

TRUAX, C. B. and MITCHELL, K. M. (1971). Research on certain therapist interpersonal skills in relation to process and outcome. In Bergin and Garfield, pp. 299–344. [200, 201, 204]

TRUAX, C. B., WARGO, D. G. and SILBER, L. D. (1966). Effects of group psychotherapy with high accurate empathy and non-possessive warmth upon female institu'tionalised delinquents. *Journal of Abnormal Psychology*, **71** (4), 267–74. [180]

TRIST, E. L. and SOFER, C. (1959). *Explorations in Group Relations*. Leicester University Press. [146]

TUCKMAN, B. W. (1965). Developmental sequence in small groups. *Psychological Bulletin*, **63**, 384–99. [78, 79, 80, 81, 82]

TUKE, H. (1892). *Dictionary of Psychological Medicine*. J. and S. Churchill. London. [85]

TURQUET, P. M. (1974a). Leadership: the individual and the group. In Gibbard, Hartmann and Mann, pp. 349–71. [64, 75, 129]

TURQUET, P. M. (1974b). Threats to identity in the large group. In Kreeger, L. (ed.), *The Large Group*. Constable, London. [132]

VON BERTALANFFY, L. (1956). General system theory. *General Systems*, **1**, 1–10. [43]

VON BERTALANFFY, L. (1962). General system theory: a critical review. *General Systems*, **7**, 1–20. [43]

VON BERTALANFFY, L. (1968). *General System Theory*. Braziller, New York. [43]

VON NEUMANN, J. and MORGENSTERN, O. (1947). *The Theory of Games and Economic Behavior*. Princeton University Press. [44]

WATSON, J. P. (1970). A repertory grid method of studying groups. *British Journal of Psychiatry*, **117**, 309–18. [205]

WATSON, J. P. (1972). Possible measures of change during group psychotherapy. *British Journal of Medical Psychology*, **45**, 71 ff. [205]

WHITAKER, C. (1965). Acting-out in family psychotherapy. In *Acting Out: Theoretical and Clinical Aspects*. Grune & Stratton, New York. [183]

WHITAKER, D. S. and LIEBERMAN, M. A. (1965). *Psychotherapy Through the Group Process*. Tavistock. London. [22, 64, 119, 135]

WHITE, R. K. and LIPPIT, R. (1960). *Autocracy and Democracy*. Harper & Row, New York. Condensed as Leader behavior and member reaction in three 'social climates' in Cartwright and Zander (1968), pp. 318–35. [60]

WHITELEY, J. S. (1970). The response of psychopaths to a therapeutic community. *British Journal of Psychiatry*, **116** (534), 517–29. [27, 30, 122, 123]

WHITELEY, J. S. (1974). The large group as a medium for sociotherapy. In Kreeger, L. (ed.), *The Large Group*. Constable, London. [139]

WHITELEY, J. S., BRIGGS, D. and TURNER, M. (1972). *Dealing with Deviants*. Hogarth Press, London. [106, 135]

WHITELEY, J. S. and ZLATIC, M. (1972). A re-appraisal of staff attitudes to the therapeutic community. *British Journal of Social Psychiatry*, **3** (2), 76–81. [127]

WHITING, J. F. and MURRAY, M. A. (1961). Toward a theory of hospital social structure based on objective data. *International Journal of Social Psychiatry*. **72**, 172–80. [93]

WHO TECHNICAL REPORT (1953). Series No. 73, Geneva. [98]

WHYTE, W. F. (1943). *Street Corner Society*. University of Chicago Press, Chicago and London. [10, 42]

WHYTE, W. F. (1967). Models for building and changing organisations. *Human Organisation*, **26** (1/2), 22–31. [141]

WIENER, N. (1948). *Cybernetics*. John Wiley, New York. [44]

WILFERT, O. (1971). Group work with offenders in institutions. *Journal of the Howard League*, **13** (2), 132–8. [179]

WILMER, H. A. (1958). Toward a definition of the therapeutic community. *American Journal of Psychiatry*, **114** (9), 824–34. [106]

WING, J. K. and BROWN, G. W. (1961). Social treatment of chronic schizophrenia: a comparative survey of three mental hospitals. *Journal of Mental Science*, **107** (450), 847–61. [88, 90]

WYNNE, LYMAN C. (1962). The study of intrafamilial alignments and splits in exploratory family therapy. Nathan, W., Ackerman, B. F. and Sandford, N. (eds), In *Exploring the Base for Family Therapy*, Sherman, New York. [182]

YABLONSKY, L. (1967). *Synanon: The Tunnel Back*. Penguin, Baltimore. [173]

YALOM, I. D. (1966). A study of group therapy drop-outs. *Archives of General Psychiatry*, **14**, 393–414. [27]

YALOM, I. D. (1970). *The Theory and Practice of Group Psychotherapy*. Basic Books, New York. [27, 33, 30]

YALOM, I. D., BROWN, S. and BLOCH, S. (1975). The written summary as a group therapy technique. *Archives of General Psychiatry*, **32**, 605–13. [37]

YALOM, I. D., HOUTS, P. S., NEWELL, G. and RAND, K. H. (1967). Preparation of patients for group psychotherapy. A controlled study. *Archives of General Psychiatry*, **17**, 416–27. [26]

ZEITLYN, B. B. (1967). The therapeutic community. Fact or fantasy. *British Journal of Psychiatry*, **113** (503), 1083–6. [105]

ZEITLYN, B. B. (1975). Group greed and group need—an occupational hazard for psychiatric personnel. *British Journal of Psychiatry*, **126**, 193–5. [126]

ZUK, G. (1967). Family therapy: formulations of a technique and its theory. *Archives of General Psychiatry*, **16**, 71–9. [183]

Index